The Invisible Pregnancy

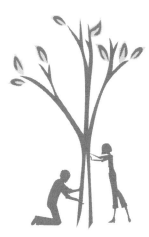

An Intimate Guide and Journal

to Mend the Space after Pregnancy and Infant Loss

"The book every midwife, doula, nurse and obstetrician should know about. It is the only sufficient guide between pregnancy and grief."

Heidi Faith CCBE CCLD SBD

With Forward by Toni *Harman,*
co-Founder, One World Birth

DEDICATION

To my family, who watched expectantly
as my grief pregnancy gestated.

To Mother Earth who carries my fourth child in her womb, and
who will one day carry my other children as well.

To Father God who tills and toils over my soul with an ancient
wisdom and deep adoration that harvests the biggest life.

CONTENTS

ACKNOWLEDGMENTS

The hundreds of thousands of families who have allowed me to walk with them to the well, have allowed me to cup their wisdom, love and truth; their tears and living water splash from their depths into this guide.
May you drink of these waters and partake of this tiny crumb of mine and may these sacraments open your soul to allow the Great Gardener to harvest that which will satisfy the hunger of your grief pregnancy.

Forward

Being pregnant is special. It is the most beautiful feeling in the world and it is a feeling that lives with you forever.

The moment you find out you are pregnant is the moment you become a mother. In carrying a baby inside you, you are connected to every other mother on the planet and to every other mother that has ever lived throughout our history as human beings.

Being pregnant is a rich spiritual universal feeling that words cannot capture. When you are pregnant, other mothers look at your growing belly and smile. They connect with you instantly.

You might have experienced this yourself, when complete strangers want to start a conversation about your baby, or ask you random questions about whether you think it's a boy or a girl or your plans for the birth. Some offer advice (often unwanted!) Some even want to reach down to touch your belly.

It's almost as though because you are pregnant, you are no longer a stranger to them. You are part of "the club" - but this club isn't exclusive. You are part of a wider global community where everyone is welcome.

I truly believe that if you are someone who has experienced loss, you are and always will be a mother. You remain part of a wider global community of mothers. You remain connected to millions of women all over the world.

That's what we are trying to do with our ONE WORLD BIRTH project. It's a global cross-media project set up by two filmmakers, myself and my long-term partner and father to our child Alex Wakeford. ONE WORLD BIRTH aims to connect individuals so that we create a global community that welcomes all.

As part of ONE WORLD BIRTH, we want to produce films and videos to help make the experience of pregnancy and birth better for all mothers around the world.

Our latest film FREEDOM FOR BIRTH hopes to raise awareness of, and ultimately bring an end to, Human Rights violations in childbirth.

We connect with these subjects because of our own difficult birth five years ago where we felt powerless and were denied choice. We knew birth didn't have to be like that.

We want to inspire a "mother's revolution" so that all mothers are afforded true informed choice in pregnancy and childbirth so that every mother is treated with dignity and respect at all times.

These are ideals we share with Invisible Pregnancy and that is why I am honoured to wrote this forward. Through the 40 Dares, the goal is to make the world a better place by helping mothers give birth to healing. It's a wonderful beautiful idea that connects with me personally as a mother and I hope will connect with you personally too.

I hope you do feel part of the wider global community and I sincerely hope that together we make the world a better place.

Toni Harman, co-Founder, One World Birth

Introduction

I was in college, rapidly advancing to become a social worker (JD/MSW), when I interrupted my own course by becoming pregnant. Interestingly, I knew I was in an unhealthy relationship at the time. In fact, I was in an unhealthy *place* at the time. As I pushed forward academically, I kept quieting that persistent voice in my heart that told me that my life was unwell. I was headed for trouble, but kept telling myself that I didn't have *time* to address it.

I knew better than this, of course. I didn't convince myself, I only ignored my Self.

I became pregnant by the man I knew I needed to leave — whom I told myself I *would* leave, eventually.

He wanted me to abort my baby. Immediately, in the very moment that I knew I was pregnant, I knew I would be a mother for the rest of my life. Growing up in foster care, every six months or so I had a new mom and dad. A new school. A new life. And while I didn't even know where I would be or what I would be doing six months from that pregnancy test, I was absolutely convinced, to my very being, that God knew. "Surely," I thought, "He would not subject my child to what I endured. He must have faith in me to gift me with this child, this person, even though I am a wreck and have no idea what I'm doing!" Telling this man that I was pregnant and receiving his response did not change this or subdue this conviction. In fact, this Cum Laude student of social work required the protection of a battered women's shelter for herself and her child. The irony is humbling.

I felt his kicks as my belly grew. I saw the ultrasounds. I experienced the contractions. But it was during birth, that I finally understood – really, understood - the marvelous discovery that his *out*sides were on my *in*side! Arms, legs, knuckles, blood and tissue were inside of me, but did not belong to me! Peculiar and awesome, life is.

I nurtured him, caressed him, fed him, and, eventually, began instructing and even disciplining him, this person, who is shaped out of me, but who isn't me. This person, this entity, who was once hidden inside me so that even I didn't know of his presence and who now, thinks outside of me, behaves outside of my expectations, decides outside of my knowledge. He isn't me, but yet was once entirely within me.

I am married now. My husband is the most courageous, protecting, committed, noble, loving, honorable, selfless man I know. To be his wife is an honor that brings me *hunting* for ways to reflect my total adoration and affection for him. We have since grown our family to include four more children, including our child who was born via miscarriage.

My first pregnancy not only brought me to my knees in surrender to the magical, powerfully redemptive work of God, but it also changed my course out of social work and into doula work, which is to come alongside other pregnant mothers and introduce them to the wisdom I had gained through my experience, and to support them – physically, emotionally, intellectually and spiritually, through theirs.

I became pregnant for the fourth time in 2011. Having the tools to support families giving birth didn't prepare me for the journey I embarked on that began in the moment I saw my lifeless baby bobbing on the ultrasound monitor. At least, *not that I was aware of.*

I looked frantically at the ultrasound monitor, expectantly believing that the God I knew would spark life, speak life, *breathe* life back into my deceased child. The ultrasound technician faded in my vision and in my mind. The walls disappeared. The only thing in my reality was the screen, was my baby. I was consumed by the presence of some strange force. I even somehow identified this fact, right there in the room. It was palpable. This presence seemed to replace the air, replace the table I lay on, replace the room I was in. I was in it. My baby and I, we were in it.

I felt this. I mean, I felt it with all of my senses, really felt it. I was terrified for my baby and for me, but was sure that everything I knew about God meant that He would bring my baby to life. I was utterly terrified, but, I had hope.

Then, the screen went black. She had shut the machine off, closed this window into my womb – into my soul – and I stared at blackness, utterly overcome.

My God was still there. But, He was silent.

I was so confused, so totally confused, I just started screaming. Right there, on the table, with cold gel on my stomach and thin paper underneath me, I started screaming at the black screen. The ultrasound technician spoke. I don't know what she said. I turned to her, and screamed at her face. The walls reappeared. I screamed at them.

My thoughts returned. I saw my husband in my mind. The father of this baby, this baby who is not alive. "He has no idea his child is dead," I thought. "I am going to have to tell my beloved that his child is dead." I screamed some more.

The ultrasound technician left the room. I slid off of the table, crumpled to the floor – trying to breathe, but the presence of an unidentifiable entity was so thick I wasn't sure if I was actually breathing. I couldn't feel the expansion of my lungs, and yet I couldn't take in any deeper of a breath.

The doctor came in, and I have no idea what she saw from the outside in. It was clear she was trying to penetrate through this force that I was encased with. She tried forcefully to plunge herself through this thickness. Her words were cold and cutting. "We need to get that debris out of there" she snapped rudely. "We need to schedule a D&C to remove it." I was horrified and humiliated, but the thickness was too big for me to digest these feelings. They simply entered into the space between us, lingering. I wailed. I needed to escape. I needed to breathe.

I called my husband.

"The baby's dead – *thebabysdeadthebabysdeadthebabysdead*" was all I could say.

I heard his voice in the receiver, and my heart melted into an even bigger mess of tears and despair. I needed to slow things down. I needed to give birth to my baby.

Over a year has passed since my baby was born via miscarriage, at home, in the presence of his mom and dad. As I have continued to support families during their birth experiences – live birth, stillbirth and miscarriage, I have come to see a poignant resemblance between grief and pregnancy, and it is my hope to reveal, in these pages, the essence of this similarity to you, so that you can begin to identify these similarities in your own life, and so that you can give birth to healing.

I have been asked so many times in the course of this journey, how I do it. How I look at so many deceased babies and the broken hearts of their parents. How I hold these things. How I do this without breaking.

This book is intended, in part, to share my answer to these questions.

I learned, somewhere in this journey, that grief is like pregnancy. I was pregnant with grief, and I needed to prepare to give birth to healing.

This book is a journal – your journal – of your grief pregnancy. It is a journey, a unique, special journey, you are on, and I am blessed to walk it with you as best I am able.

The time following pregnancy and infant loss can seem overwhelmingly empty – void of purpose, of meaning, of joy, of life. You may feel isolated, abandoned, misunderstood, trivialized, forgotten or ignored. You may feel rushed to move into some new place in your life, but you may be feeling entirely too trapped, too confused, too immobile. I believe there is a reason for this.

I believe it is because you are called to be present in this sacred space. I believe you are in a deep well of potential, like a seed planted deep in the soil. You are in a rich time that holds enormously significant potential. I believe you are pregnant with grief.

Through this book, I will invite you to explore this most sacred space, and, together we will look at this space that needs mending, that needs your presence, that needs you.

My experience with pregnancy and infant loss drew me hungrily searching for a morsel to nourish my starving spiritual Self.

There was an ancient woman, named Mary. She was a teenager, fresh and beautiful. She was betrothed to a man named Joseph. Joseph was a hard working man, a carpenter, who looked forward to completing his engagement and marrying his beautiful beloved.

Wouldn't it be, that the Great Gardener had plans that disrupted theirs? Mary was visited by an angel, and she became pregnant supernaturally.

Joseph, who was a good man, a hardworking man, did not take the news of his fiancé's pregnancy very well. Mary became pregnant out of wedlock. He didn't want to claim the child as his. He didn't want any part of what was taking place.

It took some divine intervention for Joseph to accept the situation, and accept the child as his.

The boy grew, and during his lifetime he blessed those around him – that is, he gave undeserved gifts that nourished and quenched.

Lies and rumors spread about this amazing, selfless man. Jealousy festered, and the self that grew in others wanted him dead.

On the day that his death was sentenced, his mother, heartbroken, walked along with him on the path to his death.

A faithful friend of his, walked quietly along beside her. His friend, he looked up to this man like a big brother. He had given up the life that his self worked so hard to bribe him with. As he walked along with this older woman, thoughts of devastation plagued him. What would he do now? Where would he go? What did all of this mean? Why was this happening to his friend?

The man, this selfless man, stood and bravely endured the attacks that he knew would result in his murder. His flesh being torn, he looked and he saw the total break of his mother. He looked and he saw the total break of his precious friend.

In one last gift, he called the two of them forward. He whispered hoarsely in one of his final breaths, that he wished for his mother to take his friend as his own son.

The enormity of this gift! The selflessness of this gift!

The man breathed his last, and died.

Later, quietly, the young man and the old woman, walked together to her home, heavily heartbroken over their loss.

What gift did this heroic man gift these two souls with?

I imagine the days, the weeks, the months that followed, as this gift began to open itself between these two souls. I imagine her waking, and preparing a warm breakfast, filled with love for her son, as something in her kitchen drew her to remember him as a boy, running to hide under the table. She imagined the times she leaned over him, brushing his hair out of his face, as he sat at that table reading, as a growing young man.

This other man, his friend, would enter the kitchen, yawning. He would come to her, put a thick, kind hand on her shoulder and, with a knowing look, would tell her, "Good morning".

In motherly love, she would say, "Sit down and eat; you need a good meal to start the day." The two of them would sit together at the kitchen table, both knowing they would eat and be satisfied not just of the meal, but of the rich stories the two would exchange.

She would begin by telling him stories of his friend, of her son, when he was just a boy. "I couldn't believe it," she'd say, "he just started telling the priests thing about the divine that they hadn't seen or heard before! He was teaching them!" She's let out a laugh, and he'd stare in amazement, waiting for her continue. "You should have seen their faces, John! It was true, all of it! The things he said to them were true, and they knew it!"

They'd chuckle, and then a pause, of love, of wonder, of life, would fill the space between them.

The man would speak. He would share a story about being on a boat in a storm. "Why he sent us out on the boat, I had no idea" he'd begin. "But since it was him who sent us out there, we thought we were safe! We thought that surely we were obedient and so no storm should come. The rains howled, oh how the lightning flashed! I was scared for my life! We all were!" He'd reach for a warm muffin then and break it, placing a warm morsel on his tongue before continuing. "We just didn't understand!"

Through these exchanges, Mary began to understand the sacrifice and the commitment that her newly betrothed had made, so many years before. There was something lost by Joseph, knowing that this boy wasn't entirely of his own flesh. But, through learning to mend the space, he discovered that this life he was given was much more than he had imagined.

Mary longed for her own son. Oh, how she ached for him! But he had given her this man, his friend, who had nothing, who needed a mother, and so she opened up her space after her loss and by so doing, began to discover that this life she was given was much more than she had imagined.

I did not become supernaturally pregnant with my first child, but I did become pregnant out of wedlock. The man who entered into my life who became my husband had to learn to sacrifice. He had to learn to open up the space and discover that this life, my son, that he was given, was much more than he had imagined. It is because of my first son, remember, that I even found the life of the man who died that day, Mary's son.

When I gave birth to my miscarried baby, when I looked upon his frail form and knew that I wouldn't mother him in the ways my entire being longed to, I did not see that the same man who gave a gift greater than imagined in his own last breaths was also giving me a gift of the same magnitude. It has only been in the days, the weeks, the months afterward, when I have found myself waking and shuffling into the kitchen, to prepare a warm meal, that a presence emerged, yawning, saying, "Give me a morsel to nourish me." Quietly, I would sit with this presence. Quietly, I would feed it. Ever quietly, I would listen. And quietly, it would grow, quietly, it would speak, quietly, it would nourish me. Quietly, I discovered, that I was given a life much bigger than I had imagined.

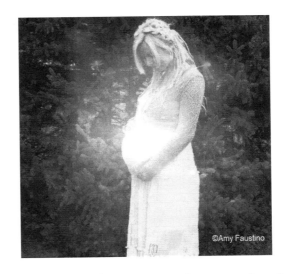

May you discover this pregnancy, and may you embrace it.

The Grief Dare

Discover your pregnancy.
Claim your labor.
Prepare for your birth.

I woke up, looked at the clock. *Twenty minutes.* I smiled, closed my eyes, and returned to sleep. Twenty minutes later, a gentle squeeze wrapped within my abdomen, around my back, and moved deep inside me. This deep pull reached below my belly button and pulled up to below my ribs. I awoke and again, looked at the glowing green light of my alarm clock: *twenty minutes.* Rubbing my belly with one hand, I stretched with my other to reach my water bottle. Bringing it to my lips, I giggled as my baby, snug within, gently stirred and bumped my hand. "We're in this together" I whisper quietly, secretly, excitedly to him. The mysterious force of labor had begun.

"Therefore keep watch, because you do not know on what day your Lord will come."
—Matthew 24:42

I labored like that, contracting every twenty minutes, for two days. The contractions were manageable, but noticeable.

On the morning of the third day, they got closer, and they got stronger.

Yawning, I reached for my soy trail mix. Chomping, I gathered fresh clothes and headed for the shower. The warm water felt nice, dripping down my body and splashing off of my round, tight belly. I began to feel more open.

After the shower, I didn't dry completely off. I let the water evaporate into my clothes as I dressed. I could feel something deep within me, something that has been closed tight since its existence, begin unlocking. I marveled at this feeling. I had been raped as a young girl. I didn't think that there was anything within me still locked in this way, and yet, I could feel it opening for the very first time. I relished in this discovery.

I felt a freedom. I locked the oven door, and used its handle to lunge into the contractions. I walked. I hummed. I sang. I chanted. I laughed. Then, I went to the hospital.

Summerlin Hospital was brand new when I was pregnant, and one nurse told me that I was the first patient she knew of there who wanted a natural birth.

Someone came into my laboring room declaring "I'm here for your scheduled water breaking." I told her to leave.

My water broke on its own – a marvelous pop! followed by the wondrous gush of warm liquid seeping into my sheets. There was a pause, and so, curiously, I bore down, ever so slightly. Immediately, the contractions thrust themselves at me, as I entered into a new realm, a place where the anticipation crosses a threshold into fruition.

A nurse could see his hair, and she invited me to touch it. I was reaching upward – my attention, was drawn upward, into the heavens. "God," I thought, "be here now." I felt as if my entire being was being ripped in two. The force, the force of my child's presence, was so big, so solid, and such an interruption to my body's physical comfort. My entire body was subject to his force, to his shape, to his destiny.

Then, his head emerged through the darkness, and I saw the most amazing person I'd ever seen in my life. The only person grown out of me. The only person I knew so intimately, and yet who was such a stranger to me. I had never seen those toes before – look at those marvelous toes! I had never seen that whorl before, and as I brought him to me, I brought his whorl to my nose and breathed deep. I gave birth.

I compare grief to pregnancy because grief is pregnancy. It begins as a result of a profound, intimate, valuable life event, and although this life event marks its beginning, we may not know of its presence until it grows large enough – until symptoms of its presence alert us to its life force, beckoning us to take notice.

It is a time in our lives that every decision we make is balanced against it. It is a season of our lives that is filled with adrenaline, fear, but also wonder and anticipation. It stirs in us a longing, a desire, an ambition, an aching, for something deep within us to finally manifest. It is a deep, intimate time of reflection, introspection, meditation, and wonder. It is a period of hidden, mysterious, and even magical growth. In its last days, a momentum drives us, the contractions of offense, hurt, disappointment, anger, abandonment, shame, all of these feelings – all of the feelings felt in grief – squeeze us until we feel we will most assuredly break in two. As the life force, this powerful entity that is of us but separate from us, bears itself out of our most intimate, darkest, deepest, most wet and raw landscapes of our very soul, finally, with sweated brows and a last long heave, we submit to this entity emerging, slippery and fragile, from the depths of our being. We can finally, for the first time, regard this thing. We meet our healing.

Now the earth was formless and empty, darkness was over the surface of the deep, and the Spirit of God was hovering over the waters. — Genesis 1:2

Like pregnancy, we don't know the exact minute it began, but we can identify the event that it was created from. You can't identify grief through two pink lines, but your body does give signs of its presence. Grief, like pregnancy, is an experience that changes us entirely. It changes our mood, the way we sleep, how we eat, and our self image.

In pregnancy, a woman is a mother. She and her child are two separate entities, and although hers encases his, the mother and the child are not the same.

While pregnant, the mother anticipates what life will be like for her once she gives birth.

Contractions come and go. They build on one another, and they move through her. The wise mother claims her response to them. She anticipates them and embraces them. She moves through them. She allows them to transform her experience and she engages in the act of labor.

In this way, the mother prepares for her birth.

Grief is the invisible pregnancy.

As you move into grief, it likely becomes apparent to those around you that it is within you. It moves. It hears you. It grows.

Like the man who told me to abort my child, feeling that your time with grief is rejected, feeling that your loved ones don't see the reality of your grief or that they don't value its potential can be enormously, profusely painful. I felt emotionally handicapped during a large portion of my first pregnancy, longing, so desiring, to have someone I love rub my belly and enter into that season of my life with me. I felt so very alone. I felt a large space of absence between myself and those around me. I felt invalidated, and in this magnificently fertile time that was awesome and amazing, I felt as if I had a profound secret – a secret, that nobody cared to hear.

I was surrounded by loving and well-intentioned people in my darkest days, but alas, I was also the recipient of the most foolish, the most insensitive, and the most mean-spirited messages. The doctor - a stranger – called my baby "debris". When I went home and called their office, a nurse told me that I "probably already flushed it". To look at my stomach, then, and not know if my body still held my baby or not, if my body had already released my child without my knowing, was flat hurtful. To be told that I was better off, that my family was better off, that this was the best thing, was meant in love, I know, but was damaging to my spirit. Then, as I shaped stillbirthday and presented this living sacrifice, to see the most ignorant accusations about my intentions – because I validate mothers – all mothers – who experience loss, that I discredit the value of obstetrics, midwifery, Christianity, and other religions, was surprising and well, annoying. The premise of this foolishness is that if I support a non-Christian mother, it means intrinsically that I do not support Christianity. The notion is absurd, and yet, occasionally, a new source of this foolishness will manifest.

Mothers bore witness to me, and would ask me how I handled these attacks against my vulnerable space of grief.

Like the pregnant mother longing to be fed a hearty meal but who is given nothing to fuel her, my core grumbled, yearning for sustenance. I would cry out in hunger, but I would not settle for consuming junk.

I believed what I needed would be provided. I believed I was being taught to find it.

I reject the messages that do not feed my soul. I do not allow these messages to be placed into my sacred space of grief. I sweep them away with a defiant brush of the spiritual broom. They are simply not allowed to enter here.

Like the pregnant mother, you need to care for your grief; nurture it, embrace it, and allow its expression. If you do not identify its reality in your life but instead try to avoid it or ignore it, it will not simply disappear. Failing to feed it and honor it will hurt it. It is within you. It is a life force. It is intended to transform you. It is up to you to decide what shape it will take. In time, and in love, you will give birth to healing.

How to use this book

This book has one intention, and that is to validate you. Your grief is a reaction of love; it is a reaction of frustration, as your desire, your longing to cultivate expression of this love feels impossibly trapped. Allowing yourself the freedom to stretch out that grief, to really open up that gap, to breathe some cleansing air into the wound of your soul, will allow you the freedom to see your grief's potential. Grief has intrusive qualities that can hurt you if you do not know what grief's value is.

Grief is valuable. It is powerful. It stretches and molds you. In your time, and with your care, it can birth into healing. Unlike a physical pregnancy, there is no force outside of you that can take it away from you. It is yours to keep, yours to nurture, yours to grow. This book is a tool to help show you how to cultivate and care for it. This book gives you permission.

Whether your experience that brought you into grief is fresh, or whether it was a long time ago, you deserve to know the fullness of the transformative labor of grief into healing. This book alone may not be enough, as is explained through the journey, and that's OK. This is only an invitation, to show you what my journey has been, and to invite you to explore your own.

This book is set up as presenting you with weekly dares. Dares are fun. As a child, it was my peers who entered into my life, came alongside it, who I felt understood me and saw me as I was, who dared me to step into a place that was a little bit scary, a little bit uncertain, a little bit new. This book is me, a peer, a fellow mother who gave birth to a deceased baby. It's me, reaching out my hand, asking to take yours, and, with a womb that carries my truth, a heart that holds my wisdom, and a twinkle of my eye that reveals my hope in you, I dare you to explore your grief with me. You can challenge yourself to each dare as rapidly or as slowly as you need. The division by weeks is only done arbitrarily, with the coincidence to forty weeks of a physical pregnancy. You will need to use your own discernment in engaging in these dares. I don't at all dare you to endanger yourself. You may feel the dares are out of order. You may feel that one was too sudden, too soon for you. It may pain you to see how I interpret my loss. I tell you these things now because you have permission to have any and all feelings that reading through my journey may bring you. These feelings grow out of an opportunity for you to claim your own journey, which may have some or even many of the same guideposts as mine, but too may be altogether different.

This book is simply my heart, telling you that you are not alone.

I have found that identifying my grief, nurturing it and then disciplining it has helped me to birth healing. I have seen it. I hold it. I want to share it with you.

In the way that no person can tell you that you are not pregnant with grief, you cannot force anyone else to claim a grief pregnancy as theirs. Someone else who has experienced loss simply may not feel pregnant with grief. If you've found this book and it has worked for you, please don't feel hurt if it doesn't work for someone you love.

As you explore the concept and the book of the Invisible Pregnancy, I recommend keeping close to a friend or two in your life who can help mentor you through this journey. This suggestion is so important you will see me mention it very often throughout our time here together.

You will need additional items to complete the dares of this book. You will need art supplies (things of your choosing, like paint, construction paper, felt, scissors, glitter, glue), old magazines, and either a pretty notebook as a companion to this book or a 3 ring binder, to include loose-leaf paper, your completed art projects, and this book (this is recommended). In the activities that ask you to treat yourself, you will need things like spa products or a little allowance to indulge the services of a professional in this area.

Giving grief a whole new perspective by comparing it to pregnancy, we have a blessed, profound opportunity to allow our grief to enrich us, to give us back something powerful that we once felt was robbed of us. We have the gift to nourish our grief into healing.

Heidi Faith

Could I possibly be?
I try to peer into my soul to see if it will reveal
any indication to me.
I hear the words for the first time, and
something stirs from within.

Am I pregnant with grief?

20

___ DARE 1

A mother's birth story is very important and powerful to her. It is her account, of her own life events. It is her interpretation. It may not be her complete assimilation of the experience, but her documented thoughts can in fact help her to begin to assimilate what is a monumental event in her life.

Going back, what was the event that propelled you into grief?

Was it the birth of your deceased child?

If your baby had a difficult diagnosis, did you experience "anticipatory grief" while still pregnant? How did this impact your birthing plans?

Maybe your event was hearing the confirmation from a medical professional that you are infertile.

Perhaps there doesn't seem to be an initial event, but just a slow, mysterious deepening.

What was the event that initiated your grief?

Spend some time this week with those initial feelings; journal about the birth of your baby.

Preparation

Choose a private place where you feel comfortable and will have no interruptions (turn off your phone, and let others know not to disturb you).

Set aside enough time to do the activity so you do not feel rushed.

Plan to do something relaxing or enjoyable after you have finished the activity.

Try to relax (slow breathing) and clear your mind of other concerns before starting the activity.

The Dare

You can type or handwrite, depending on your preference.

Do not be concerned with spelling, grammar, or punctuation.

Write your account in the first person (use "I" statements).

Write your account in the present tense (as if it is happening right now).

Include as much sensory detail as possible (sights, sounds, smells, textures, etc.)

Include any thoughts and feelings you had at the time.

Even though it may be painful, do not stop yourself from feeling emotions.

Keep writing until your account is complete, even if this takes a while.

Feeling Safe

Try not to stop halfway through to process a specific memory. Keep working through it if at all possible.

Remind yourself that this is just a memory and that you are in a safe place.

If you become overly stressed, you can choose to take a brief break from writing, but should continue as soon as possible.

Identify a couple of strategies that will help you to feel safe and reduce anxious feelings (slow breathing, having a glass of water).

Identify two people you can contact immediately if you need help.

When You are Finished

Take time to congratulate yourself on revisiting these feelings.

Treat yourself to something relaxing or enjoyable.

Your invisible pregnancy is only just beginning.

Heidi Faith

Your Sacred Space

__ DARE 2

This week, take yourself back a little further.

Go into your pregnancy, when you were pregnant with your child.

Where were you, emotionally? Where were you, spiritually?

What fears did you have? What dreams did you have?

What words would describe you then? Trusting? Blissful? Unsuspecting?

Who were you, when you were pregnant?

Let's get a little messy this week – literally. Get out the paint, and brush and smear a beautiful portrait of your time in pregnancy.

Preparation

Choose a private place where you feel comfortable and will have no interruptions (turn off your phone, and let others know not to disturb you).

Set aside enough time to do the activity so you do not feel rushed.

Plan to do something relaxing or enjoyable after you have finished the activity.

Try to relax (slow breathing) and clear your mind of other concerns before starting the activity.

The Dare

You can use the art supplies of your preference.

Do not be concerned with technical features.

Capture the experience in the first person (how you envision yourself through your mind's eye, or, of what you saw through your own lens).

As you craft your piece, bring your memory into the present tense (as if it is happening right now).

Include as much sensory detail as possible (sights, sounds, smells, textures, etc.)

Include any colors, strokes or shapes that represent thoughts and feelings you had at the time.

Even though it may be painful, do not stop yourself from feeling emotions.

Keep working until your piece is complete, even if this takes a while.

Feeling Safe

Try not to stop halfway through to process a specific memory. Keep working through it if at all possible.

Remind yourself that this is just a memory and that you are in a safe place.

If you become overly stressed, you can choose to take a brief break, but should continue as soon as possible.

Identify a couple of strategies that will help you to feel safe and reduce anxious feelings (slow breathing, having a glass of water).

Identify two people you can contact immediately if you need help.

When You are Finished

Take time to congratulate yourself on revisiting these feelings.

Treat yourself to something relaxing or enjoyable.

Name your piece. There is a special power in claiming this piece as yours, and of gifting your work with a name. Add this work into your Grief Dare portfolio or binder. If it is very large, snap a photo of it to include in your journal.

The magic of her wonder is still within you.

Your Sacred Space

__ DARE 3

This week, return to Dare 1.

Review your written account, and highlight or underline any "hotspots" in it. These are areas of particularly intense emotion.

When you are finished, go through your work again, observing the hotspots you have chosen. On a fresh sheet in your journal, list each one, and journal the urgency you feel, if any, in challenging each of them.

Brave to look at your pain.

This moment was hurtful. Very hurtful. It hurts just to look at it. I don't have to fix it today, but, today, can I whisper to myself the knowledge that I have a power within this pain?

Preparation

Choose a private place where you feel comfortable and will have no interruptions (turn off your phone, and let others know not to disturb you).

Set aside enough time to do the activity so you do not feel rushed.

Plan to do something relaxing or enjoyable after you have finished the activity.

Try to relax (slow breathing) and clear your mind of other concerns before starting the activity.

The Dare

You can type or handwrite, depending on your preference.

Do not be concerned with spelling, grammar, or punctuation.

Write your account in the first person (use "I" statements).

Write your account in the present tense (as if it is happening right now).

Include as much sensory detail as possible (sights, sounds, smells, textures, etc.)

Include any thoughts and feelings you had at the time.

Even though it may be painful, do not stop yourself from feeling emotions.

Keep writing until your account is complete, even if this takes a while.

Feeling Safe

Try not to stop halfway through to process a specific memory. Keep working through it if at all possible.

Remind yourself that this is just a memory and that you are in a safe place.

If you become overly stressed, you can choose to take a brief break, but should continue as soon as possible.

Identify a couple of strategies that will help you to feel safe and reduce anxious feelings (slow breathing, having a glass of water).

Identify two people you can contact immediately if you need help.

When You are Finished

Take time to congratulate yourself on revisiting these feelings.

Treat yourself to something relaxing or enjoyable.

Like the tiny seed of a tree,

or the precious embryo of life,

you are growing a truth, deep within you.

Your Sacred Space

__ DARE 4

You now have a list of "hotspots" – a specific listing of the most devastating moments, captured, side by side, together.

This list, looking at it, makes even the paper it is written on feel heavier.

It's hurtful.

It's sad.

Let it in.

For this exercise, you have your list, of the deepest offenses. You've spent some time with them. Now, it's time to look at them with your thinking, logical, evaluating mind.

Preparation

Choose a private place where you feel comfortable and will have no interruptions (turn off your phone, and let others know not to disturb you).

Set aside enough time to do the activity so you do not feel rushed.

Plan to do something relaxing or enjoyable after you have finished the activity.

Try to relax (slow breathing) and clear your mind of other concerns before starting the activity.

The Dare

You can type or handwrite, depending on your preference.

Do not be concerned with spelling, grammar, or punctuation.

Reflect on one hotspot at a time.

Identify and journal on why you think this hotspot is distressing to you.

Search your spirit. Can you identify any unhelpful core beliefs or thinking styles you may have carried through this hotspot?

Search honestly and deeply. Are there any alternative and less distressing ways of viewing this hotspot? You are journaling only, not applying any action or change right now.

Even though it may be painful, do not stop yourself from feeling emotions.

Keep writing until your thoughts are complete, even if this takes a while.

Feeling Safe

Try not to stop halfway through to process a specific memory. Keep working through it if at all possible.

Remind yourself that this is just a memory and that you are in a safe place.

If you become overly stressed, you can choose to take a brief break, but should continue as soon as possible.

Identify a couple of strategies that will help you to feel safe and reduce anxious feelings (slow breathing, having a glass of water).

Identify two people you can contact immediately if you need help.

When You are Finished

Take time to congratulate yourself on revisiting these feelings.

Treat yourself to something relaxing or enjoyable.

Let it out.

Your Sacred Space

Heidi Faith

__ DARE 5

For this week, you should have chosen at least one (and, only one is absolutely fine), of your hotspots to re-phrase in a non-emotional way.

Allow yourself this week to hold this new interpretation.

Conjure feelings of compassion, mercy, gentleness and forgiveness toward your offender. Maybe it was someone who said something utterly thoughtless to you. Perhaps it was the lack of support you felt – maybe, you felt abandoned and minimized by people who hold a large presence in your life. It is possible that you have been angry or ashamed at yourself for losing this baby. Or, you might be disappointed in the God you thought you knew.

Instead, speaking the truth in love, we will grow to become in every respect the mature body of him who is the head, that is, Christ. –Ephesians 4:15

Forgiveness doesn't mean to forget. Gentleness doesn't mean to dismiss the reality. The reality is that you have felt wounded. You can hold your experience, and allow your thoughts to shift from being problem, emotional and past- based, to being resolution, intellectual and future- based. You can engage in your healing. You can speak the truth – but, you can speak it in love. This week, allow your grief to challenge you to enter into love; to feel only love, to come alongside the offender in love, if even only in your mind's eye, to rewrite the reasons for their actions.

41

Replace your defensive reasons that are from your perspective, with the loving reasons from theirs.

Patiently enter their witness.

Preparation

Choose a private place where you feel comfortable and will have no interruptions (turn off your phone, and let others know not to disturb you).

Set aside enough time to do the activity so you do not feel rushed.

Plan to do something relaxing or enjoyable after you have finished the activity.

Try to relax (slow breathing) and clear your mind of other concerns before starting the activity.

The Dare

You can type or handwrite, depending on your preference.

Do not be concerned with spelling, grammar, or punctuation.

This is only a time of journaling. You do not need to encounter any past offender.

Search your spirit. Can you identify any other reason for their action other than one that is intentionally cruel and predatorial toward you?

If you cannot identify one loving reason for their action, be still. Calmly accept that their loving reason simply eludes you. In times like this, I remember that the person was blindsighted, used, taken advantage of by a cruel force. I remember that my perpetrator is a victim of this force, just as I feel the victim of this person. As I transform from victim – someone who is defined by hurt – to a survivor – someone who is victorious over the feelings that victimization once brought – I have empathy for my perpetrator, my aggressor, the victim.

Search honestly and deeply. You are journaling only, not applying any action or change right now. He or she need not know of this searching.

Even though it may be painful, do not stop yourself from feeling emotions.

Keep writing until your thoughts are complete, even if this takes a while.

Feeling Safe

Try not to stop halfway through to process a specific memory. Keep working through it if at all possible.

Remind yourself that this is just a memory and that you are in a safe place.

If you become overly stressed, you can choose to take a brief break, but should continue as soon as possible.

Identify a couple of strategies that will help you to feel safe and reduce anxious feelings (slow breathing, having a glass of water).

Identify two people you can contact immediately if you need help.

When You are Finished

Take time to congratulate yourself on revisiting these feelings.

Treat yourself to something relaxing or enjoyable.

Your witness does not lose value
by exploring theirs.

Your Sacred Space

Heidi Faith

__ DARE 6

This week, your dare is to relax.

Relax.

Preparation

Choose a private place where you feel comfortable and will have no interruptions (turn off your phone, and let others know not to disturb you).

Set aside enough time to do the activity so you do not feel rushed.

The Dare

Observe the way you feel physically and mentally, before and after each relaxation exercise. Journal these reactions, to allow you to see the effects over time of practicing relaxation.

As you journal, note what emotions you are feeling.

What thoughts were going through your mind?

Because tension levels build up over time, you may not be accustomed to recognizing when your body is tense and when it is relaxed. That's OK; we're going to labor through this, together.

Read through the following instructions once, so that you know what you will be doing. Then bring these instructions near you so that you can follow them along while remaining in your comfortable position. This activity should take 15-20 minutes:

In your private, quiet place, either sit or lie down with your arms and legs uncrossed, with spine aligned, in a comfortable position.

Gently close your eyes, or let them rest on a single point in front of you.

Take a slow, deep breath, in and out from the belly.
Take another, a little deeper this time.

You may feel your body start to relax and let go.

We're going to work through our body, from head to toe, tensing and relaxing muscle groups.

Start by creating tension in your upper face.

By scrunching your eyes tight shut and frowning, holding the tension.
Now, letting go of the tension, letting your face relax, you're noticing the difference between tension and relaxation.

This time, create tension in your lower face, by clenching your jaw, with a fake smile on your face.

Holding…

Letting go, noticing the difference between tension and relaxation.

Hold the tension in your shoulders and neck, shoulders up and neck in – holding.

Letting go, relax and feel the tension release. Let your shoulders drop and chin release – how much better it feels to let go.

Bend both elbows and tense arms. Push your shoulders back and chest out. Your arms may quiver with tension.

Let your tension go. Let the relaxed feeling spread throughout your body.

Slowly make a fist with both hands. Observe the tightness in your hands and arms as you squeeze. Letting go of the tension, uncurl your fingers.

Feeling more, and more relaxed.

Tighten your stomach muscles, making your stomach as tight as you can – hold the tension.

Relax your stomach muscles, letting go of tension.

Take in a slow deep breath to let go of any remaining tension. Tighten and flex the muscles in your lower back and buttox – holding the tension.

Let go, and relax.

Let your hips relax.

Feel completely and deeply relaxed.

Hold the tension in your upper legs – hold the tension, keeping the muscles tight.

Let go, notice the difference between tension and relaxation. Relax.

Push your toes down, away from your body, holding the tension in your lower legs. Notice what the tension feels like.

Letting go...

Feel the heaviness spread throughout your body as you relax, deeper still.

Arche your feet, push your arches up, toes down.

Relax.

Letting go of any remaining tension. Notice the feeling of relaxation spreading through your entire body, from your head to your toes.

Enjoy the feeling for several minutes.

Let your attention flow to your effortless ebb and flow of breathing in and out of your body.

Feeling relaxed, but gradually more alert. Gently moving your toes and fingers.

When you are ready, open your eyes and give your body a wake up stretch, feeling awake and relaxed.

When You are Finished

Remember to journal your feelings when you are finished.

Repeat this practice every day this week. Each time, it should take you approximately 15-20 minutes to complete. You will come back to this dare many more times – as you commit to doing this entirely and completely, it will take progressively less time. It will eventually become a tool you can use at any time of day, in any place, wherever you need it.

You are awake and relaxed.

Your Sacred Space

__ DARE 7

This week, we are going to reflect on dare two.

Go back into your pregnancy, when you were pregnant with your child.

Study the art piece you made. Speak its name aloud. Touch your work.

Now, what do you feel is lost, was taken away, or is gone now, that you experienced pregnancy loss?

From the past, to the present, and into the future, call those things into your mind that are not what you thought or hoped for.

Claim the space.

Let's get a little messy this week – literally. Get out the paint, and brush and smear and show a vivid look into this space.

Preparation

Choose a private place where you feel comfortable and will have no interruptions (turn off your phone, and let others know not to disturb you).

Set aside enough time to do the activity so you do not feel rushed.

Plan to do something relaxing or enjoyable after you have finished the activity.

Try to relax (slow breathing) and clear your mind of other concerns before starting the activity.

The Dare

You can use the art supplies of your preference.

Do not be concerned with technical features.

Capture the experience in the first person (how you envision yourself through your mind's eye, or, of what you have seen through your own lens).

As you craft your piece, bring your memory and your thoughts into the present tense (as if it is happening right now).

Include as much sensory detail as possible (sights, sounds, smells, textures, etc.)

Include any colors, strokes or shapes that represent thoughts and feelings you have.

Even though it may be painful, do not stop yourself from feeling emotions.

Keep working until your piece is complete, even if this takes a while.

Feeling Safe

Try not to stop halfway through to process a specific memory. Keep working through it if at all possible.

Remind yourself that this is just a memory, just your thoughts and feelings, and that you are in a safe place.

If you become overly stressed, you can choose to take a brief break, but should continue as soon as possible.

Identify a couple of strategies that will help you to feel safe and reduce anxious feelings (slow breathing, having a glass of water).

Identify two people you can contact immediately if you need help.

When You are Finished

Take time to congratulate yourself on revisiting these feelings.

Treat yourself to something relaxing or enjoyable.

Name your piece. There is a special power in claiming this piece as yours, and of gifting your work with a name. Add this work into your Grief Dare portfolio or binder. If it is very large, snap a photo of it to include in your journal.

I paint with jagged strokes of frustration, downward brushes of disappointment, curving inward in my shame; I then grab the liquid symbolism with my bare hands – I feel a force within me telling me I need to feel this – and I clump it into my canvas, pushing, pushing it deep, so the paper weakens under the pressure. The color is so thick it drips down my fingers, onto the floor. As I use the back of my hand to wipe my tears from my face, I smear sticky color onto my cheeks. I feel like a tribal, warrior princess.
This is the ultrasound of my grief.

Your power is alive.

Your Sacred Space

__ DARE 8

This week, we are going to have some directed journaling.

Take a calm stroll around your soul.

Get out your journal, and take time to really consider the questions posed to you here.

Preparation

Choose a private place where you feel comfortable and will have no interruptions (turn off your phone, and let others know not to disturb you).

Set aside enough time to do the activity so you do not feel rushed.

Plan to do something relaxing or enjoyable after you have finished the activity.

Try to relax (slow breathing) and clear your mind of other concerns before starting the activity.

The Dare

You can type or handwrite, depending on your preference.

Do not be concerned with spelling, grammar, or punctuation.

Keep writing until your thoughts are complete, even if this takes a while.

Journal your answers to the following seven questions:

What do I currently do to relax?

What have I done in the past to relax (in childhood or adulthood)?

What does enjoyment mean to me?

What are some examples of activities I would find enjoyable?

What makes me laugh?

What are some activities I can plan to do (at least three)?

How can I incorporate these activities into my life?

As you contemplate, take note of any intrusive thoughts or images, and if there is anyone or anything you avoid as a result.

This is purely a journaling exercise; you do not need to act or engage in these activities at this time.

When You are Finished

Take time to congratulate yourself on revisiting these feelings.

Treat yourself to something relaxing or enjoyable.

All those things you've always wanted to do...

...you should go do them.

Heidi Faith

Your Sacred Space

__ DARE 9

This week, our alarm clocks may get involved in our work.

I am opening up my morning, opening up my day,

I am opening up my thoughts.

Whatever time you usually wake up in the morning, I am challenging you now, to wake up one hour earlier. So get out the trusty alarm clock if you need to, because this dare is going to be good. Like many of these dares, I encourage you to consider allowing this to become a new ritual that becomes a part of your daily life, not just during this week.

Preparation

Set your alarm clock if you need to. Perhaps the best way to start this dare is to go to bed one hour earl

Choose a private place where you feel comfortable and will have no interruptions (turn off your phone, and let others know not to disturb you).

Set aside enough time to do the activity so you do not feel rushed.

Plan to do something relaxing or enjoyable after you have finished the activity.

Try to relax (slow breathing) and clear your mind of other concerns before starting the activity.

The Dare

Waking up early seems such a painful thought, at least to me, anyway. I treasure my dreams, my warm, comfortable time when I don't have to serve anybody else but can bask in the warmth of nothingness.

This early morning time holds so much potential, so much fertile growth of our souls, if we just allow it to feed us.

Staying in your pajamas, your warm socks and slippers, wrap a warm robe around your body and let the belt hug your belly securely. Shuffle into the kitchen. Start a pot of coffee, if you desire. Let the strange, lovely sounds of the water boiling and cooking into the fresh ground beans delight your ears. If it's tea that you enjoy, marvel at the whistle of the kettle as the air in the water, otherwise quiet, squeals with delight as it pushes out of the toasty container to tell you that your water is ready to meet your delicious pouch of leaves. Perhaps your delight is hot cocoa. As the cold milk splashes into the shallow pot, study the thousands of tiny bubbles that rise from the bottom. See how the froth moves to hug the center of this pool of white as its temperature changes from cool to warm. As the waves of evaporation increase, you know that the milk is thickening ever so slightly as it warms. It is ready to steep the sweet powder of rich, dark cocoa.

Wrap your hands around the cup that holds your morning hot broth of invigoration and peace.

Look out your window now. Drink up the sights of the sky, the tops of the trees, the houses of your neighbors, and of your yard, of bushes, of branches, of grass. Note to yourself any crispness, any coldness, any budding of life, any caressing of colors and any boldness or subtlety of presence in any of these things.

Then, taking your warm drink, and maybe even a snack if desired, go into your quiet place with your journal.

For the remainder of this hour, you are going to spend time with your grief.

You are going to just spend this time, communicating and speaking to your grief.

You can choose if you will do this by directing your attention to your grief as a listening, responding entity, or if you will do this by directing your attention to your child; if you desire to direct this activity toward your child, you will need to remind yourself that your child is not you, your child is not the culmination of your wishes, but that your child is his own entity, with his own life force, with his own destiny and purpose. It is cruel to discredit and devalue his purpose by only sending him complaints about your own lack of vision.

Talk right out loud, if you can, without disturbing anyone else in your home.

If you can, without disturbing anyone else, perhaps put on some music and dance or act your expressions, letting your body movements tell the story of your desires, your wishes, your longings, your hopes, your growth, and your journey.

Alternatively, if you are too concerned with waking someone up in your home, whisper these things aloud.

Whisper, and acknowledge to your grief the thoughts that go through your mind. Tell it your longings, your disappointments, your dreams, your wishes. Tell your child the things you've experienced, things you've learned, things you wanted him to experience and things you wanted him to learn.

Then, when you are finished, be still.

Be quiet.

Wait.

In your heart, search for a response. You will hear one, if you wait. If you are open. If you are patient.

Who is it you are hearing from?

For me, I hear both from myself, and my Self. I hear myself telling my Self that I am a plumb fool for talking out loud. It mocks me. It tries to shame me. I hear my Self tell myself that I have permission to do this, to grow. That the mockery grows only because I'm on to something that I am afraid of, but that I'm OK. I'm safe. I have permission.

I listen.

I call out the things myself try to show me: fear, shame, self consciousness, and doubt. And in my mind's eye, I show it the darkness that has grown around me and that I've allowed to enter into me. I show it my anger, my temper tantrums, my outbursts, my lowered limit of tolerance, acceptance, and grace. And I ask it, "Which is better, this ugliness, or, this foolishness? This ugliness has to go. I am making room in this place for healing."

And then it quiets.

I can return to waiting and listening.

I become aware of a sacred presence in my stillness.

I bask in it, in this time alone, with just me, and my thoughts.

When you have finished in this time of talking outwardly and of listening inwardly, journal your experience, and your feelings. Look out your window once again, and note how the world has changed since your sacred, intimate time.

Now, commit the remainder of the day to think of anything other than your child. As thoughts of your child enter into your mind throughout the day, look at them, identify them, and then give them permission to float away. You have already committed your energy to your child this morning. You've indulged in intentional presence with your grief. You can let these thoughts go.

You will do this activity again tomorrow – right now, this thought has permission – has *instruction* to leave.

My Self tells me when a thought is intrusive.
I listen.
I have permission to take every thought
captive and make it obedient to my indwelled
Self.

Your Sacred Space

___ DARE 10

This week, we are going to enter into our minds.

This is my own, familiar, foreign place.

For this activity, you will need a special book; for me, it is my Bible. We will read until we meet a special message, and then we will carry this message with us, and journal on it.

Like many of these dares, you may repeat this one fresh with a new message each day.

You may enjoy doing this as an extension of week nine's dare, doing this immediately after your time of what I call prayer, of being active and of being still in sacred presence.

Preparation

Choose a private place where you feel comfortable and will have no interruptions (turn off your phone, and let others know not to disturb you).

Set aside enough time to do the activity so you do not feel rushed. You will be reading until you find treasure – give yourself at least an hour. This is a great morning activity.

Plan to do something relaxing or enjoyable after you have finished the activity.

Try to relax (slow breathing) and clear your mind of other concerns before starting the activity.

The Dare

You can type or handwrite, depending on your preference.

Do not be concerned with spelling, grammar, or punctuation.

Keep writing until your thoughts are complete, even if this takes a while.

My favorite way to do this activity is to start by holding a mantra. In order to hold a mantra, however, we first must gather one.

The best place for me to find mantras is in Scripture. Maybe you have your own very special book of truths, or other writing filled with love and inspiration. Whatever your book, get it out. Rub your hand across its cover. Feel the texture of the material, of the print of the title. Open your book, open it, and burrow your nose into the crease between two pages, breathing in the culminated smell of paper, ink, glue and binding. Breathe the aroma. Is it of dust and ancient wisdom? Is it of crisp fresh revelations? Both? In your comfortable place this week, let this book invite you in.

This is not a race; this is not a competition or an activity to merely check off in accomplishment. You do not need to start at the very beginning, unless you simply want to. You do not have to read for a set period of time, and you do not have to read until you've reached a certain page. Just, simply read.

Read, as an archeologist. Read, digging, until you find something. How will you know when you've found something? You'll feel a prompting. Like the archeologist feeling a sudden bump! meeting his efforts, you will feel a gentle but firm prompting as you first meet with what is to be your mantra. Then, you'll get out the dry, clean brushes, push back the loose dirt around this thing. You'll get out your picks and scrape away some more around it. You'll get out your camera and walk around this piece, snapping pictures and feeling both satisfied that you've found it, and enthralled in wonder at what this small revelation can possibly be connected to. "What else is under there?" you wonder.

Of course, all of this is just a metaphor. You aren't digging this week. This week, you're reading. Reading, until you find something. It will be something small. For me, it's a Bible verse. I read, until a verse prompts a feeling within me that lets me know I struck something. Maybe I finish the story, and then return to this verse, or maybe I stop right there. Either way, I am careful with this treasure – I don't overlook it, I don't race past it to accomplish reading. The archeologist's mission isn't to dig as deep a hole as possible, but he is willing to dig as deep a hole as necessary to find his treasure. Your time in reading for this activity may be short, or it may be long, but your reading should be slow, patient, and deep. You should be open, listening, waiting to find the treasure.

Once you've found your treasure, write it down.

Write it in your journal. Then, spend some time with this message. Read it on your paper. See how it looks in your own handwriting. In your quiet place, be alone with this message. Allow it to bring images into your mind. Allow it to bring thoughts into your mind.

As other thoughts enter in, distracting, unrelated thoughts, look at them. Identify them. Then, gently allow them to fade away. In this way, this slow, quiet, gentle way, you are inviting your mind to only think of your special message, and clearing your mind of any other thoughts.

Ask your special message questions. Put it into scenes in your mind's eye, playing a game with your message. Allow it to communicate with you, showing you what it is that it is trying to show you. Laugh with it. Cry with it. Be curious and open with it.

Journal the thoughts you have about your special verse or your special phrase you've been given.

Then, write your verse again, this time on a scrap piece of paper – maybe you'll rip a page out of your journal, or maybe you'll use some other paper. Either way, rewrite your verse onto this paper. Stick it in your pocket. Carry it with you throughout the day. Each time you have a moment to let your thoughts wander, open up this paper and read your message, and bring your thoughts back to this verse.

This verse is your mantra.

Last week we began claiming our thoughts. We are learning how to mother our minds. We are cradling our minds, nesting in the home of our thinking, removing the clutter that keeps our mental home stagnant and ill, and opening up space for healing. This week, as you continue to identify disruptive thoughts, and as you continue to gently let them go, replace them with your special message.

Your special message, your mantra, was given to you for this purpose.

Hold it, carry it, and let it speak to you.

The God who holds my baby is not so far away.

He is here, speaking to me. I quiet myself to listen.

Heidi Faith

Your Sacred Space

__ DARE 11

This week, we are going to enter the outside world.

This place is ancient and worn, yet undiscovered.

We're going to go back to dare eight – the dare where you looked at some enjoyable things you might do. This week, we are going to start putting action to those thoughts, by beginning to envision yourself engaging in one of your chosen activities. But first, we're going to get outside to do a different activity – one that I dare you to.

Preparation

Choose a private place outdoors where you feel comfortable and will have no interruptions.

Set aside enough time to do the activity so you do not feel rushed.

The Dare

Dress appropriately for the weather to keep yourself comfortable and healthy. This activity is best on a warm, sunny day, but any weather will do.

Choose a place that will likely have few other people around or other distractions such as loud traffic. A beautiful, scenic garden, an untamed prairie, a beach, or even your own back yard can all work well.

In this place, stand comfortably, spine aligned, arms gently dropped to your sides.

Breathe.

Bring the air of this beautiful place into your being; deep, into your being.

Exhale tension, doubt, and any negativity.

Breathe in deep, again.

Notice your body receiving this cleansing air. Feel your body digesting it, moving its loveliness into your arms, your fingers, your legs, all the way down to your toes.

Feel the warmth of this freshness fill your heart.

Just simply stand, breathe, and look.

Weather permitting, find a terrain that will be gentle on your bare feet, and take your shoes and socks off.
Feel each blade of grass bend beneath your weight.

Step forward, slowly.

Capture everything you can about this place, about this

experience.

Breathe. Feel your breath.

Walk. Feel your steps.

Listen – really listen, intently, to what you are hearing.

This is a very slow, methodical, exploration of this place.

As disruptive thoughts come, identify them, and then gently let them drift off. If they return, identify them again, and again, simply let them gently drift off. They will leave.

Be present. Be only here.

When you have finished exploring, journal your experience.

You can type or handwrite, depending on your preference. If you'd like, you can find a quiet, soft place to sit, and continue to explore this place as you journal.

Do not be concerned with spelling, grammar, or punctuation.

Keep writing until your thoughts are complete, even if this takes a while.

When You are Finished

Consider expanding on this activity by repeating it on another day, this time holding your mantra, and in the stillness, being open to receive any messages, clues or answers that your mantra may be inviting you to find. I believe that God's goodness is in everything, and that clues to His loving message to me can be found wherever I'm at. Don't limit your communication with your grief – just like a pregnant mother, you carry it with you wherever you go. You may be surprised at how it longs to reveal a message of love to you.

As you've chosen one activity that can bring you enjoyment, begin today to take steps to make this activity come to fruition. Maybe you want to take up sewing, and your first step is in finding a beginner's class. Maybe it's riding a hot air balloon or baking or jogging. Go to the shoe store then, or schedule savings into your budget for the items you will need.

Your grief speaks the language of the Earth to reach your soul and prepare you for healing.

Heidi Faith

Your Sacred Space

__ DARE 12

This week, we are going to look at nutrition.

What are you allowing to enter into your body? What fuel are you giving yourself to work, to cleanse, to grow your grief into healing? What message are you sending to yourself, by what you place into your body? Are you gifting and nurturing yourself, or are you shoving toxins and forcing emptiness into yourself as some form of contempt for your vessel?

I am valuable,

and what I consume will reflect this.

Begin to plan a healthy menu. The right foods will help your grief grow in the way it needs to. The right foods will help you grow in the ways you need to.

I erroneously believed once, that grief is something that should be kept small and silent.

I was wrong.

It shouldn't be explosive, nor should it be destructive, and left unchecked, grief has the dangerous potential to be these things. But my grief is something to treasure. It's something that, if given the right sort of space, direction, and handling, can and does manifest into something magnificent. I am not afraid of my grief. I feed it, whether I realize it or not. I will be intentional with what I feed it. If I feed it only healthy things, than it will grow and transform in a healthy way.

The best foods for your soul are the foods that still speak the Earth language the clearest: raw, fresh from the Earth's table.

Your dare this week is not only to begin to plan a healthy menu every day of the week, but to use food as a communicator of health and love for your husband.

Your husband is valuable. He should too, only be consuming the best foods that reflect this. Your dare isn't to totally uproot your regular meal planning, but to show him that you love him through one, planned, lovely, intentional meal.

In fact, pick his favorite dish.

Add fresh veggies or a salad as a first course, present him with his favorite dish as the main course, and use your creativity for things like side dishes, bread, drink and dessert.

The Dare

Part 1: Begin to prepare a menu that welcomes health and healing.
Part 2: Prepare a loving meal for your husband.

As you plan the meal for your husband, plan it to be as lovely, beautiful, romantic, and special as you can. Maybe this means pulling out the nicest dishes. Getting the nicest cut of meat. Preparing a meal as extravagant as Thanksgiving dinner. Using a nice tablecloth, and decorating the table with flowers or candles.

I have done this activity several times and is one of my most favorite ways of telling my man I love him.

One way I have done this, is to prepare a nice hearty roast in the crockpot. This frees me to make sure everything else is in place when he comes home from work.

Then I bring a low, wide table into the living room, that I can plug the crockpot into. I move the couch out of the way and lay big, heavy blankets on the floor, in front of our fireplace, and toss some lighter ones on top of them, with some pillows. I bring in a cooler, fill it with ice and a bottle of champagne. I write a card that says that I love him – that I simply love him, and I lay it on the blankets for him to find.

Have fun with this dare. As you plan your grocery list and the items you need, do it without telling him. I hope this dare finds you giggling with excitement.

On the day that you complete this dare, free your mind from any expectation you have of him in his reaction. Don't shove your surprise on him as soon as he walks in the door from work. Let him discover your process and, in behavior and in attitude, simply invite him to step into the experience with you.

As you eat, practice the skills you learned on your walk, in how to really be present: chew your bites slowly, really savoring the flavors of your meal. As your mouth fills with the zest, the flavors of your husband's favorite dish, fill your heart with love and adoration of him. In this way, it is not you sharing a meal with him, but you are allowing him to share this meal with you.

When You are Finished

After the meal has ended, journal on the experience. What healthy foods did you pair with his favorite dish? Fresh bread? Veggie sticks as an appetizer? A healthy dip? Dessert?

In your journaling, begin to dedicate space simply listing the things you are thankful for in your man. From the trivial things, to things of long ago, to daily things in your lives, begin to look for, find, and identify these things. Write them as they come to you, and give yourself plenty of space in your journal to add to this list in the weeks ahead.

My man has grief too.
I am the mother. I know now that my
man is silently turning to me, waiting for me to
nurture this grief inside of me into healing.
As my most inner Self grows and becomes
evident, he will take notice and he will take part.

Heidi Faith

Your Sacred Space

__ DARE 13

This week, I am calling you to the most intimate act of love.

Make, love.

Love is something you can make. Like the way we eat, we can put emptiness inside of us, or we can be totally enraptured with a pure, refreshing sustenance that quenches our deepest thirst.

Preparation

We ended the dare last week by beginning to create a thankfulness section of our journal. We have begun looking for things in our spouse that we are thankful for. You will need to begin working on this portion of your journal in order to complete this dare. Maybe you'll leave a couple of blank pages before your pick up your writing on other subjects, or maybe you can reserve a special portion of your journal.

Maybe, you'll just add a paragraph each day into your journal, to include the things you've discovered in that day, of what you are thankful for in your man.

However you decide to do it, it is extremely important that you have begun to write this growing list.

The Dare

You are going to initiate physical intimacy with your spouse. You should decide to make this dare as exotic, as passionate, and as lovely as you can. You might want to plan ahead on how you will prepare this activity.

I for one have issues – many – with physical intimacy. I was raped as a little girl. I was always the tallest and the most flat-chested girl I knew, which I allowed to feel left out. I didn't have strong parents to help shape my identity. I gave birth to a miscarried baby. All of these things taunt my self image, and require the lovingkindness of my Self to protect me, to correct and even discipline the many untruths these things speak to me.

I would begin this dare with some careful self examination. Get in front of the mirror. Let the clothes that shield you drop from your body. As you release each one, look at the parts of your body they covered, they protected, that they even hid. Caress them, ever so gently, just letting your hands softly stroke your skin. It's just you here. You are alone. You are safe.

Get to know yourself, through the lens of your Self.

Your arms are valuable. They carry and hold things. They hug. They hold up. See your arms. Look at them. Look at any freckles you may have on them. See the soft hairs. Look at the creases in your elbows. Begin to admire your arms, for how capable they are, for how beautiful and valuable they are.

Do this, complete this activity, giving a good long look at your entire body. Look at your face. Look at your beautiful, lovely face. It is lovely.

As you do this activity, remember to identify any negative thoughts, and gently let them go. They are not welcome here. This is your body, your sacred space. Tell them to go, and they will flee from you. I say this, because the negative thoughts will come. And they are not true.

They will come to you now, because they are not true. Because your self is selfish and doesn't want to lose you to your Self.

Look at your face. Look into your eyes. See the gentle bend of your eyelashes. Keep looking. See the curves of your ears, and the beautiful movement of your head, the gorgeous turn of your eyes in order to do so. A slight, mysterious, beautiful glance.

I am beautiful.

Tell yourself that you are beautiful.

Smile. And, say it again.

Identify which parts of yourself are most difficult to believe are lovely. Let your Self linger over those parts longer. As you speak love into these parts, ask if any of them have to do with the pregnancy of your child. How was your baby born? This may too, impact your view, may tempt you to denounce your worth.

If your baby was born with additional medical assistance, for example. Needing a D&C can be emotionally painful. Perhaps you had an emergency Cesarean birth, and now bare the scar where your baby emerged, and it may feel as if this strong, tender skin is the entryway into a dark, hidden tunnel, a place of constant sorrow.

Our innermost wounds heal when we look at them with a discipline to grow and we touch them with a tenderness to guide them into growth. For example, a mother who has given birth to a child previously through Cesarean, can have her uterus gently but firmly massaged where it bares the mark of her child's passage. This massaging can help increase her likelihood of then giving birth to a subsequent child vaginally. Additionally, a massage technique called pelvic floor massage is a practice of intentional touching to bring release from the depths of a woman's most intimate of physical places. This is not only a service that some professionals do offer, but it is something that you have the right to explore for yourself. This is not to be mistaken for perineal stretching, which is a technique that does also include rubbing but for the purpose of preparing the vagina's thin outer skin for the stretch that may happen during childbirth. Pelvic floor massage, at first blush, seems nothing more than masturbation. The thought of masturbation brings me to shame, as my childhood days of innocence were ripped from me, and as I long to be faithful to what I know of my God, I do not want to displease my man by taking away an opportunity he would otherwise have at quenching both of our physical desires.

I say all of this, because palpating your own pelvic floor, or allowing your husband to do this, is a wonderful way of simply exploring the space. Of getting to know the terrain of your secret place. The intention is of being present, within, and fulfilling this intention brings a release that secondarily, can bring with it eroticism and even orgasm. It is not out of shame, but rather out of reverence of my own most authentic Self, that I tell you that getting to know this place myself, and/or allowing my husband to, would only magnify this experience, and that at the hands of a stranger, albeit a professional one, would, for me, retract from this intimate and profound experience.

After you have spent this time alone with yourself, speaking love messages to your parts, regions and places, take time to journal your feelings.

Was this a difficult assignment? Did you stop?

I have allowed the beauty of modesty to hide my shame, shame that needed to be looked at closely with an eye of discipline and of nurturing. Examine the messages you hear during this activity, between your self and your Self.

Is this activity something you hear your Self telling you that you can and should do again?

Now, you will plan how you want to present yourself – your

93

Self – to your husband.

As you've grown in this journey, I think that a slow revelation is best.

To begin, I might prepare a warm foot soak for him as he comes home from work. I give him the first ten to fifteen minutes after he comes home, to just be home: to take his shoes off, to hang his coat up, to use the restroom. Then, I invite him to a comfortable chair, where a cool glass of water or his favorite drink may be (this might be a soda, beer, or something else, whatever his favorite is).

Perhaps you might decide to have on some makeup, and maybe even a special outfit to wear as you wash his feet – something that indicates what your intentions are for the evening.

However you want to plan this evening, is up to you, based on what you know your husband's desires to be, and how you are willing to dare yourself to challenge your own insecurities and even your hurts.

Believe that your man wants the gift of you.

The most important part of this dare, is to recall your list of things you are thankful for in your man. As you rub his tired feet, or as you draw your fingernails down his bare back, your every action during this activity should be to express your thankfulness for him. Speak this thankfulness silently to your legs, and let them fall open to receiving him. Speak this thankfulness silently to your fingers, and let them tighten their grasp on him.

If you hold a wound that you feel is too deep for intercourse, remember that looking at it with discipline to grow and touching it with a tenderness to guide it, will shape it into the healing it longs for. Ignoring this wound will not heal it.

Perhaps this is a dare that will need to be moved into very

slowly for you. Remember, each mother's grief pregnancy is different. Rushing through it won't help it grow well. Starting off with an evening of simply laying together, spending time touching one another, may be what is best. Tell him that this is what your intention is. Make it exciting, adventurous, and invigorating.

This is an act of full presence, of full participation, of full surrender, of full communion.

My God! I love this man!

Your Sacred Space

__ DARE 14

For this dare, you will need to find a tree. You will need to select a tree, in a special place.

Weather permitting, you can choose from variations of this dare, including drawing or painting a tree.

The first part of this dare makes a mess. The second part places order.

My child has a place in history.

My child has a place in the future.

My child has a place in the present.

My baby was buried. His physical form remains in the tomb – his womb of the earth, until the great manifestation of the spiritual awakening called the Rapture.

Preparation

Find a special tree in a quiet place, where you can work on this activity with little interruption. A secluded park, an old forest, or a tree in your back yard would work well.

Bring a gardening tool; whatever you may have (hoe, rake, shovel or even just a spoon) to break the dirt. You will also need a container of water.

The Dare

I look at my family tree, what I know of it. I was taken from my mother at a very early age, and was taken from my father after I was abused. I draw from my birth certificate and the moments in my relationship with my parents when they spoke of their histories. I piece together the ancestry, my heritage. It is a family I have loathed yet have longed for, a family that knew me but a moment but have impacted me profoundly. I carry the truth of my family lineage in the freckles on my skin and the predispositions to certain illnesses within me. I hold an unknown wisdom of painful lessons and beautiful victories.

I hold my family tree, the notes I have written. Birth dates, marriages, deaths. The tree becomes knotty, warped, twisted and misshapen by multiple divorces. The distorted web of branches is to me a secret code that hides and yet reveals bouts of drunkenness, domestic violence, perverted lusts and undisciplined desires.

As I place myself within this tree, this tree that humbles me, I place my deceased child in his proper place as well. I mark his presence in my heart. In my life. In the universe.

How many of my ancestral mothers didn't do this?

How many of them buried the reality of their child?

My child's physical form is buried in the depths of the earth. There are many possibilities that can have happened in your experience. Perhaps your baby was too small to identify for certain, and for you, flushing was the process of delivering his physical form into our waterways, where it is transformed by the creatures of the sea, and through the water cycle and through photosynthesis, it still carries a meaningful, powerful life force. Being buried as ashes, whether individually or collectively, as some hospitals offer for example, still does not change this power. Contemplate these things as you read my exploration of the power of my child's physical form.

His tomb is really a womb, where the process of decomposition creates a heat, and this heat becomes a hearth for the creatures who reside below my feet. These creatures are drawn to the warmth of this transformation. They are pulled, instinctively, to this magical change. They crave it. My baby's physical form draws them near to it, in the way I am drawn to gazing into a fire. These creatures, they taste of it. It nourishes them and satisfies their desires. It cares for them. It nurtures them and fills them where they hunger. When they are filled, they move away, satisfied in a way they hadn't been before.

As the process of digestion takes place, their bodies release hints of my baby's majesty as a trail of greatness. The infinitesimal seeds of grass that reside in the soil see these morsels through the eyes of their tiny roots. They excitedly reach, stretching their roots, stretching to reach these treasured nuggets of life. Finally, a root reaches a precious, microscopic bead of this creature's digestion, and it relishes it. It embraces it. The reality of my child nourishes the grass. It bursts through the darkness and it captures my adoring gaze. I reach down to pat the soft grass.

I go to where my child is buried, where just below my feet I know these magical events are taking place. I scoop some of this dirt, and place it in a jar. I carry this magical mystery home with me. My child's life feeds the earth.

Mother Earth holds in her womb my child. She swells as my child grows and changes more of the world than I can possibly imagine. I feel infinitely humbled to know that I am this child's mother. He is of me, but is not me! He is moving forward, in life. This truth admonishes me to use my own arms, my own mind, my own skills and my own abilities to impact the world for good as well. This is the body I have been given, to communicate good, to nourish others and fill them with warmth and delight.

As a baby emerges from the womb, a warm, almost hot water is released. As I look into my soul and see my pregnancy of grief growing, there is a warmth in my soul. Dear God, give me eyes to see how this warmth can bring joy! Show me how it can satisfy!

I go to my special tree, the tree I have chosen. I sprinkle this special dirt at her feet. I pour water into the dirt.

I reach my hands into the spreading river of life.

I swirl. I squish.

I make patterns, long lines, loops and curvy lines.

I allow my mind to sway, as branches sway to the pulls of the wind. I simply allow myself to enjoy playing in the mud.

Barefoot, I squish my toes into the mushy mess, painting my feet brown.

As I play, I think of my family tree. I think of the strong women before me, who carried invisible pregnancies. I imagine their force, their strength, as today, our invisible pregnancies still are not identified and cared for the way they should be. These lonely, courageous women. These lonely, courageous men, who fathered these invisible pregnancies. The unspoken forces of distension and disorder growing between couples who didn't see the invisible force of grief that could grow them together. I see the families who could have been, if only they gave birth to healing. I sadden as I see how they allowed the power of their grief to turn into something dangerous and hurtful, and how my predispositions to certain illnesses is because these microscopic morsels of their undisciplined and unloved grief have been passed down into my body. I cry over the invisible pregnancies of my ancestors, and I beg the Eternal Healer to begin to birth healing out of these ancient, forsaken cells of grief.

My fingers move into the mud, tracing the lines of pleasure on Mother Earths face that this secret has been discovered and that this healing is birthing. She smiles at me, winking, as she passes down the unspoken secrets of my ancestors. This wet mess enters my pours, the life in this message enters my soul. I will carry forward this truth. I will be a part of making a clearer family tree for the generations after me. For my own children, for my cousins, for my nieces.

This place, this is where my child is added to my family tree.
When I am done playing, contemplating and swirling, I stand back and admire this strange, messy, message of pain and of healing.

When you are finished, snap a photo of your artwork at the base of the tree. Paste or tape this photo into your journal.

For the second part of this dare, you are invited to create a family tree for your child. In truth, your child may or may not be present in your official family tree or if you have a special format (some families have birth stones on a placard or some other significant representation), your child's place may not be marked. Let that be OK, if that is to be.

Here, in your journal, you will make your own map of ancestry, and it will include your child.

My child, I carry you with me.

Family Tree

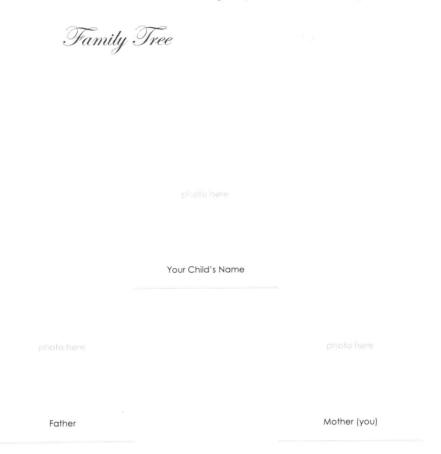

Your Child's Name

Father

Mother (you)

Your Heritage

Write about your parents' families. Describe what you remember about your parents, your grandparents, aunts and uncles, and other relatives. Talk to family members to get more information. It doesn't matter how you organize the information. This is your book, and you can write it any way you like.

Dad

If your husband has written his life story, type or copy it here. A lot of what makes you who you are comes from your parents, so your husband's story is also your child's story.

If you have pictures to go with your stories, insert them as appropriate.

Mom

If you have written her life story, type or copy it here. A lot of what makes you who you are comes from your parents, so your story is also your child's story.

If you have pictures to go with your stories, insert them as appropriate.

Courtship & Marriage

Spend time reflecting and journaling on how you and your husband met, courted, and married. Tell the story with all of the little details, and then include it in this section.

If you have pictures to go with your stories, insert them as appropriate.

Your Brothers & Sisters

Use this section to journal the fun times you dreamed of your children sharing, and of the special, enjoyable, important ways you mother your living children.

Medical History

The more you know about the medical history of your ancestors, the easier it is for doctors to diagnose health problems that you might have. Particularly if you believe that your medical history may be linked to your experience, you may want to include this section in your child's special family tree. Remember, you hold the truth of your invisible pregnancy, and you can leave pieces, clues, behind that can make it easier for mothers after you who carry their invisible pregnancies to find their truth.

Name of Person

(Illness, Surgery or Other Event) (Date) (Description)

(Invisible Pregnancy) (Dates to Know) (Important Events)

Family Traditions - With You

Use this section to write about the things that your family does, specifically to hold the intentional space of your child in the family. This may include visiting the headstone where he is buried, or taking a trip to a fish hatchery as you reflect on the life force of your child entering into our water system, as the grass that lives because of him is then consumed by livestock and birds, and then the release that they bring is washed into waterways by the gentle carry of raindrops. Maybe your special tradition is throwing a special stone, perhaps with a lovely word or symbol inscribed on it, into a nearby river, pond, ocean, or brook.

Perhaps you release a balloon or bake a cake on his stillbirthday. "Placenta" means "cake" in Latin. If your pregnancy loss was a blighted ovum, a cake might become especially significant and validating to you.

Write about the traditions you have, why they are important, how they got started, and any other information you'd like to include.

If you haven't created any special traditions, use this space to consider creating one.

If you have pictures to go with your stories, insert them as appropriate.

Family Traditions - Without You

You are not forsaking your deceased child by relishing in the joys of your life. Whether you have living children or not, you are right to engage in events and traditions that bring meaning and beauty to your life. You do not need to intentionally create a space for your child's reality in everything you do, In the way a living child eventually stretches, matures, and moves away from his mother, your deceased child's reality, too, needs space to move into the fulfillment of his purposes. His life force is moving, it is bringing health and life to the world. You do not need to dwell in what you believe he is missing or what you believe you are missing. This in fact blocks the potential for the fullness of his life. Treasure in the times you have released the intentional space and have just filled it with your own joy and your own life.

These traditions and events can include special holiday activities, trips you take regularly, yearly visits to relatives, religious ceremonies, and so on. Use this section to write about the things that your family does regularly and that are important to you.

Add a heading for each tradition. Write about the tradition and why it is important, how it got started, and any other information you would like to include. If you have pictures to go with your stories, insert them as appropriate.

Heirlooms

Journal about the heirlooms you desired to pass down to your child, what special items you've collected from your child, and what you imagine you might do with these special items someday. Will you pass them down to someone you love?

Your Sacred Space

Heidi Faith

__ DARE 15

In this dare, you are going to create an online video.

Standing at the threshold of this place,

waiting for another mother to step forward,

I clasp her hand and whisper,

"Let me show you what I've learned."

Preparation

Getting familiar with movie making tools will be very helpful. Here are the following:

Web-Based Animoto: http://animoto.com/

Movie Maker for PC: http://windows.microsoft.com/is-IS/windows-live/movie-maker-get-started

For Mac: http://www.apple.com/ilife/imovie/

The Dare

You can choose which scenario you want to film:

You are a nurse or maybe an ultrasound technician to a mother who is just discovering her grief, her invisible pregnancy, and you are giving her useful information.

You are a travel agent, giving a little brochure to mothers who are newly embarking on the journey of grief.

You are an older sister who is pregnant with grief, and your little sister has just discovered that she too, is pregnant with grief. You share with her what you've experienced so far, knowing you are still pregnant, you haven't yet given birth to healing and so you know you have more to learn, but that you have gained true wisdom and deep insight that is valuable to share.

Your video will be filled with encouragement. It should be a beautiful, lovely welcoming into this mysterious journey of the invisible pregnancy. It can be a little fun, or silly, too.

Your video must include your journal in some way. Perhaps you will video record yourself holding your journal and turning the pages. Maybe you will use one or more of the photos you have taken, or you will read an excerpt from your journaling. Maybe you'll speak one of your mantras or will use them as captions in your video.

Your video can be a collection of photos and captions that move with a special song, it can be entirely one segment of video recording, or it can be a combination. The creativity of this is yours.

Your video must be somewhere between four and seven minutes long.

When You are Finished

When your video is created, please add it to the stillbirthday collection of Invisible Pregnancy videos at
http://www.stillbirthday.com/invisible-pregnancy

I carry a mysterious wisdom.
It is mysterious even to me,
even though I know it is within me.
A valuable life force that is growing into
healing is implanted in my soul.

Heidi Faith

Your Sacred Space

___ DARE 16

This week we're going to go back to dare eleven, and ask some questions.

Have I moved beyond intention?

In week eleven, we explored the space outdoors. We also allowed ourselves to imagine activities we might engage in that can bring us joy or pleasure. You should have put into motion the first steps necessary to bring one activity into your life, whether it was to purchase running shoes or register for a beginner's class.

How are these steps completed at this point?

This week, we're going to journal some of our thoughts about these activities, about the one in particular we selected. If you haven't yet begun any active movement into the activity you selected, we're going to take a gentle look at the possibility of it holding some tension or even fear for you. If you have begun your activity, we're going to look at any possible stresses you may encounter during your activity. What sources of conflict could arise by your engaging in your chosen activity?

In the end, we are also going to review these questions in a whole other angle – through the lens of your work on dare five.

Preparation

Choose a private place where you feel comfortable and will have no interruptions (turn off your phone, and let others know not to disturb you).

Set aside enough time to do the activity so you do not feel rushed.

Plan to do something relaxing or enjoyable after you have finished the activity.

Try to relax (slow breathing) and clear your mind of other concerns before starting the activity.

The Dare

Reflecting first on the chosen activity you selected for week eleven, answer the following:

Preparing for your activity:
What is it that I have to do?
What is the real likelihood of something bad happening?
Have I done this successfully before?
What is the benefit of seeing this situation through?
Do I have a plan to deal with this situation?
What coping strategies can I use to help me face stress presented in the situation?

Preparing for feelings:

What can I do to feel calm if something in the situation creates stress?
What techniques can I draw from: breathing, progressive muscle relaxation, staying present?

Reviewing the activity:

How did I handle any stressful moments in the situation?
What can I do differently next time?
What did I do well?

Now, turn back to your dare five, the one where we spent some quiet time meditating on a new, different way to view any one of the offenses we may have encountered. Sister, let me tell you, I have encountered some offenses since I became pregnant with grief, and I know you have too. I know this journaling is a difficult one, but I am daring you to prepare your heart for an actual encounter with the person you selected for dare five. Calling this person into your mind, I'd like you to go through these questions you just looked at, and answer them in accordance to a meeting with this person.

You can type or handwrite, depending on your preference.

Do not be concerned with spelling, grammar, or punctuation.

Write your account in the first person (use "I" statements).

Write your account in the present tense (as if it is happening right now).

Include as much sensory detail as possible (sights, sounds, smells, textures, etc.)

Include any thoughts and feelings you had at the time.

Even though it may be painful, do not stop yourself from feeling emotions.

Keep writing until your account is complete, even if this takes a while.

Feeling Safe

Try not to stop halfway through to process a specific memory. Keep working through it if at all possible.

Remind yourself that this is just a memory and that you are in a safe place.

If you become overly stressed, you can choose to take a brief break from writing, but should continue as soon as possible.

Identify a couple of strategies that will help you to feel safe and reduce anxious feelings (slow breathing, having a glass of water).

Identify two people you can contact immediately if you need help.

When You are Finished

Take time to congratulate yourself on revisiting these feelings.

Treat yourself to something relaxing or enjoyable.

I make allowance in my journey for setbacks.

I acknowledge and I maintain my gains.

Your Sacred Space

__ DARE 17

What gender does your grief resemble?

I hold my belly, which once held my child.
This place now holds my grief, and it is
expanding.
It is taking on a shape I never imagined.
I look to this place, and I ask this force
within, "What gender are you?"

Preparation

Choose a private place where you feel comfortable and will have no interruptions (turn off your phone, and let others know not to disturb you).

Set aside enough time to do the activity so you do not feel rushed.

Plan to do something relaxing or enjoyable after you have finished the activity.

Try to relax (slow breathing) and clear your mind of other concerns before starting the activity.

The Dare

Reflecting on your behaviors, attitudes, and decisions since becoming pregnant with grief, determine which gender your grief has taken.

Your grief may look very similar to your previous responses to frustrations, disappointments and hurts, or it may look entirely different.

When I was a little girl, I learned to pick up on a sense of the winds changing. I could feel the tremors of change before the storm of dissatisfaction and imperfection would displace me into another stranger's home. I responded immaturely, that is to say, I didn't respond in a way that would make sense to any witnesses. Simply put, I broke my things. I would take my dolls, any favorite barrettes or trinkets or any other things I might have had, and I would destroy them. Shatter them. Crumple them. Trash them. I would slam them into the trash receptacle with a broken satisfaction that I had control over what anyone else could take away from me.

This was an emotional, female response. Not to say that women or girls respond this way, or that anything that seems illogical is emotional and everything emotional is female. But the response was one rooted in my feelings, nothing else. I felt I had control, and I silenced the voice of my Self who told me

127

otherwise.

When I felt that heaviness in my heart in the ultrasound room, knowing I would have to tell my husband that his child was dead, my soul felt as if it broke all over the room, filling it with broken bits of heartbreak. Each step, each moment, only crushed me further. I was so ashamed to have to tell him. I felt like I wounded him to the depths of possibility.

It is both the love for my child and the love for my husband that crafted my grief. In spending time evaluating, looking at and being still with my grief, I discovered that it resembles a masculine life force.

I didn't crumple and hide my grief. I didn't take it away. I told my entire community of farmers that I would need to borrow from their very best gardening tools. This life force needed some serious pruning, watering, and sunshine. I held within me, a broken tree, and I needed to tend to this thing.

I needed to mend the space.

So, the community of farmers I called upon brought up their shovels, they brought their picks, their plows, their watering cans.

Many of the tools were unuseful. The words given to me cut too deep, or they were ineffective, or they didn't work properly. Some were designed for other life forces, and simply didn't work with what I had.

Somehow, just identifying the need to find the right tools, gave this life force a bit of what it needed.

Occasionally, when I felt it was right, I would display this creation for my man to witness. I tried to do this tenderly, because in our marriage, he is the farmer, the strong gardener. I was broken for him, because I knew this creation was just much too strange, much too difficult, for him to cultivate, shape and care for by himself. In the earliest days, I believe he didn't want me to notice this life force, because he didn't want to break me with knowing it was too much for him to care for himself.

Oh, in those earliest days, when holding this creation was so new to us. How we each wanted to hide it so that the other didn't have to see! I recall how it scratched us both, so that we each were so busy mending our own hurts that we failed to see the potential for this thing to become something beautiful.

I remember when we didn't know the sacred power of grief.

I discovered it first, I think, or at least I think I was the one who spoke of it first. I had secretly been pruning, silently been watering, caring for this, my grief pregnancy. I tended to it in a way that was very new to me, a way in which I realized had a great many masculine qualities.

Use these indicators below, and meditate on your grief pregnancy. Journal your thoughts and feelings on the style and life your grief is resembling.

Female:

Intuitive grievers feel grief intensely and find expressing emotions by talking or crying is helpful.

They are comfortable with expressing strong emotions, are sensitive to their feelings, and are aware of the feelings of others.

Sharing feelings about the loss and providing support to others can be very healing for the intuitive griever.

Identifies others as source of support.

Openly expresses feelings.

Temporarily withdraws from responsibilities.

Allows time to experience inner pain.

Joins support groups.

Chooses ways to express feelings – journal, quilt or other project.

Male:

Instrumental grievers experience grief, but it is less intense or emotional and more physical than the intuitive griever.

Instrumental grievers like to think or problem solve ways of coping with the experience.

For instrumental grievers, the grief tends to be more private or hidden.

They might be reluctant to talk about their feelings.

Masculine, versus conventional, grievers, shelve thoughts and feelings to cope with the present.

Masculine grievers choose active ways of expressing grief, such as hobbies.

Uses humor to express feelings and manage anger.

Seeks companionship.

Uses solitude to reflect and adapt.

Writes or journals.

Did you notice that this list doesn't seem extremely definitive? It is because it requires you to be still, to be present with your grief.

You can learn some things about your grief from others or from me, but you will need to be still, be present, with your grief, in order to learn from your grief.

As you meditate on your grief and as you allow yourself to enter into a sacred space with it, journal on your thoughts relating to the gender of your grief.

You can type or handwrite, depending on your preference.

Do not be concerned with spelling, grammar, or punctuation.

Write your account in the first person (use "I" statements).

Write your account in the present tense (as if it is happening right now).

Include as much sensory detail as possible (sights, sounds, smells, textures, etc.)

Include any thoughts and feelings you had at the time.

Even though it may be painful, do not stop yourself from feeling emotions.

Keep writing until your account is complete, even if this takes a while.

When You are Finished

Take time to congratulate yourself on revisiting these feelings.

Treat yourself to something relaxing or enjoyable.

Dear mysterious force,
I am learning who you are.
I am learning your potential.
I am learning your power.

Your Sacred Space

Heidi Faith

__ DARE 18

This week's dare is to spend time with your grief, and then journal your experience.

I am learning you.

Learning what your grief is, is really painful, challenging, invigorating work.

Deep into my grief pregnancy now, I recall the darkest days and enter them into my own Invisible Pregnancy journal:

The implantation bleeding of my grief began in the restroom, as I returned home from the ultrasound office and the encounter – the intrusion – of the doctor's harsh words. The most impossible experience became etched into my mind's eye. The most hopeless of realities became mine. Alone, in the restroom, it was as though my body could finally exhale, it finally having permission to weep its crimson tears of sorrow that my child had died, now that I had heard the truth. My body waited for my mind to know. How weak my mind must have been, I wonder, that it needed this gift. It is a gift, nevertheless, I remind myself. I stir a little, with annoyance maybe, or perhaps it's a wince, as I sit in my quiet, safe place. I notice this. "Hush," I tell my legs as

134

they shift, "I am safe here."

My husband looked at me, deeply, expectantly, curiously. I looked into his glistening eyes and entered a well, where I fell, wonderfully, fearfully fell into a warm pool of the deepest love I had ever seen. This entryway hadn't seemed here before, I remember noting. It seemed as if something in his soul had broken, and had released this hidden pathway into his depths. I was so ashamed of this breaking, I felt so broken for him, the father of this child whom I felt so responsible for. The space between us and around us was filled with the heaviness of the newness of grief. I felt responsible for this heaviness, since it was my discovery that led us to feeling it. And yet, in my humility, in my smallness, I felt so entirely enamored by this deep well of love I saw in my man, standing, strong and courageous before me. I felt my soul plunge into the warm pool of his love. I needed him then, and I let myself need him. In this strange new land, he was what I knew.

As you transform spiritually,

your physical form can become more

vulnerable.

I see this, I know this, of pregnancy. I know this of the magical, mysterious time of gestation. As a child is knit in my womb, I feel the Creator enter into His Creation, filling it with His consuming attention and love. How frail a baby is! How vulnerable a pregnant mother is! Her immune system weakens. She becomes more easily weary, fatigued. Nausea, constipation, heartburn, swelling, a sense of unbalance. Pregnant mothers need to treat their bodies with care, because of the deep spiritual transformation they encounter simply by knowing a seed has been planted. Moms of all religious backgrounds have proclaimed, exclaimed! the spiritual work of the Holy Spirit within their laboring temple.

I know that being pregnant with grief has brought me into a deep, spiritual place, and it continues to. As my soul deepens, my physical form becomes more vulnerable.

I have felt physically weak. Incapable. Tired. Taxed. Too

quick to allow junk into my body and into my soul.

Jesus spoke with a woman like me. She was tired. She felt overburdened. She allowed junk into her body and into her soul.

He walked with His disciples through Samaria. They reached a well, and, Jesus told the men that He was tired and hungry, and He sat at the well. The men left to go buy food.

A woman arrived, and, as she dipped her bucket to gather water, He asked her if she would give Him a drink. I ponder this, Divinity asking of humanity. Whatever spiritual beliefs you have, imagine your God stooping down to ask you to serve and satisfy Him. The thought is marvelous to me!

They had a conversation, she and He. She seemed to scoff at Him, surprised this foreign man was speaking to her. She must have really been surprised when He offered her living water!

"Whoever drinks the water I give them will never thirst. Indeed, the water I give them will become in them a spring of water welling up to eternal life." –John 4:13&14

Oh, how I identify my self in her reply:

"Sir, give me this water so that I won't get thirsty and have to keep coming here to draw water." –John 4:15

I have wanted the right thing, for the wrong reason.

It is only when I am face to face with the Truth that I do not have this thing, that I am able to, embarrassingly, shamefully, whisper this Truth.

Jesus responded by telling her to go and get her husband. She didn't have a husband. She didn't revere her body as a holy temple and only allow that to enter her which would grow her Self. She allowed junk to enter. She allowed men to enter her, men who had not first entered into a covenantial committed relationship with her.

Jesus, breathe life back into my child!

"Go, bring back to me the selfless and Self ful reasons why I should fulfill this request" He replied into my soul. I could argue, and protest, and compile a pretty convincing argument in my self's defense. But, I knew better. I know that once in my life, He could have given me anything but a child, but He chose to give me my beautiful son, and it was through that gift that I came to follow Him. Now, years later, when I meet Him again, I expect Him to do the same. He didn't. I was called to learn more about Him.

The woman was so entirely moved by this experience, by Jesus really witnessing her, that she left her bucket with Him and ran into the town to tell everyone about the Great Messiah.

She left her bucket with Him.

She was once weary to even gather her simple provision. The thought of gathering water didn't quench her, but was instead a burden. She was a woman in a town full of people who knew her emptiness. She allowed men to misuse her well and take from it until she felt empty. While pregnant with grief, I too have walked within my community and have felt the stares, the judgment, the displacement. She is a woman like me.

What I marvel at in this interaction, is that when the disciples return, Jesus rises to His feet, refreshed, yet He hadn't eaten yet.

What I capture from this encounter is that the Divine was nourished by quenching her spiritual thirst, and in so doing, promised to impregnate her with a life force that will manifest into eternal life!

"Whoever drinks the water I give them will never thirst. Indeed, the water I give them will become in them a spring of water welling up to eternal life." —John 4:13&14

I remember what I know to be the immediate and rapid transformation of my child's physical form in the womb of Mother Earth. I envision the creatures, the feeding, the releasing, the water cycle. Then I imagine a spring of water within me, welling, up to eternal life. His physicality is changing and sustaining the earth. His spirituality is changing and sustaining me.

I am learning that giving life isn't what I once thought it meant. My grief pregnancy is calling me to a fresh awareness and a renewed service, to participate in the life around me.

This is my mantra.

My grief pregnancy is becoming in me a spring of water welling up to eternal life. My child's spiritual life is eternal. So is mine.

I realize that other mothers are on a treck up to their well. They are unsuspecting mothers who will endure pregnancy loss. I tremble in tears as I know they are stepping closer to that place where they will first encounter their self, and I speak to the Jesus who waits there, quietly for them, feeling wounded for them but knowing what He will offer them. They will leave their buckets with Him, and they will go

I whisper to Him, "Please, can I sit with You, and meet her here too?"

Grief is transforming into a gift. My grief pregnancy is a splendid, spiritual awakening. It is not a deficit. My grief hearkens me to lean into the warmth of the Divine.

Yet I remember the little girl of my youth, and I too easily call into my mind young ladies I know who were thrust into motherhood, the hymenal shedding that pierced through their bodies through the force of rape and which began physical pregnancies became for them the implantation bleeding of grief. These women who found the implantation of a child within them to be an offense that was too intricately connected to the robbery of flesh and spirit they survived.

To these women, the only way they could heave their weary

bodies forward to carry their meager bucket to the well was if the seed of pregnancy was carved out from them.

Motherhood is not grown into the fullest potential it can be by every mother, and yet these mothers in my memory still hold the same opportunity to have a Divine encounter, and they too, have the same opportunity to birth healing from their grief journey. My child's spiritual life is eternal, with or without my consent or my participation. My spiritual life is too, eternal, and I can birth healing and run to give life back into my community, or I can eternally shuffle, alone, broken, in darkness, miserly seeking that which will not nourish me. Similarly, I ponder, just how not every physical coitus results in physical pregnancy, not every loss impregnates a mother with grief, and not every grief pregnancy is identified, nurtured and disciplined to give birth to healing. And even those who are, we will still have special differences in our pregnancies, things that make our own experiences unique. I contemplate these things, as I am pregnant with grief, and it is moving me closer toward the day I meet my healing.

The woman left her pail with Him.

This image enthralls me. I dwell on it.

She complained about needing to carry it to the well, and yet left holding more water than she thought possible. She had become a well.

Can I lay my pail at Jesus' feet? Can I give my God the things I have, the things I need? Could I see two pink lines and give the outcome of the pregnancy over to Him?

Could I believe that the celebration of my communion with my husband could bring forth a different sort of life? A different kind of pail?

Pail.

Pregnancy and Infant Loss. I find this such a unifying acrostic. I lost a pregnancy *and* an infant. I can identify the point in my child's life in which he died: he died during pregnancy.

I met my God's presence at the discovery of my pregnancy

and infant loss – when it was identified.

Can I lay my PAIL at His feet? What implications does this have for me?

I am being Divinized.

As I meditate on and journal these things, I invite you now to meet with your own grief pregnancy.

Preparation

Choose a private place where you feel comfortable and will have no interruptions (turn off your phone, and let others know not to disturb you).

Set aside enough time to do the activity so you do not feel rushed.

Plan to do something relaxing or enjoyable after you have finished the activity.

Try to relax (slow breathing) and clear your mind of other concerns before starting the activity.

The Dare

One of the best ways to really get into this dare is to draw from the exercise of dare nine, where you were first called to be intentionally present in the space. If that hasn't become routine for you, consider picking it back up this week and establishing it as part of your daily ritual.

As you enter into the powerful stillness, meditate on your grief.

Call into your mind how it first began.

Call into your mind how it behaved in the earliest days, when you hadn't yet articulated that you were pregnant with grief.

Draw into your vision the journey it has brought you on.

Are there any dares that you know need to be repeated or completed? What about the dare to eat more healthy food? To have deeper intimacy with your man? How are yoru daily mantras enriching you? Did you stop looking for them after the dare was over? Have you used Progressive Muscle Relaxation lately? Have you looked upon yourself in love?

Contemplate where you believe your grief may be leading you, what it may be preparing you for. Your grief should be leading you into a place that is new and that can seem scary, but a place that reveals the biggest version of your Self.

Evaluate honestly the quality of nurturing you have given your grief.

Evaluate honestly the quality of discipline you have given your grief.

You can type or handwrite, depending on your preference.

Do not be concerned with spelling, grammar, or punctuation.

Write your account in the first person (use "I" statements).

Write your account in the present tense (as if it is happening right now).

Include as much sensory detail as possible (sights, sounds, smells, textures, etc.)

Include any thoughts and feelings you had at the time.

Even though it may be painful, do not stop yourself from feeling emotions.

Keep writing until your account is complete, even if this takes a while.

When You are Finished

Take time to congratulate yourself on revisiting these feelings.

Treat yourself to something relaxing or enjoyable.

*Her grief pregnancy was identified.
It was nurtured in respect and validation in
her conversation with the Divine.
Then it was disciplined as she went back into
her community to face the people who only
previously saw her darkness. She reached into
their lives. She spoke to them. The spring of
life burst and refreshed.
She met healing.*

Your Sacred Space

Heidi Faith

__ DARE 19

This week, we are going to look at our connections.

I am part of a community.
In my grief pregnancy, I can and will
commune.

Years ago, people used to stop by one another's house for tea. This was so commonplace, many would even come over unannounced.

How many visitors have you had come knock on your door in recent months? How many times have you gotten together with your girlfriends and just been present together? This week, we're going to look at the need to get connected.

Preparation

What are you sharing with your husband about your grief pregnancy? How engaged are you in your social life? Do you have friends? When is the last time you and your husband went out on a date, or your girlfriends gathered together to giggle?

Prepare for this dare by first contemplating on your connections.

The Dare

This dare has two parts.

For the first part, you are going to be intentional in your daily connections. Make eye contact with the bank teller, read the name tag in the check-out line at the grocery store, and thank the cashier by name. Reach out and make one form of physical contact with your spouse every day, whether it's a hug, pat on the back, placing your hand on his cheek, resting in his arms, or placing your hand in his. Every day this week, engage in physical contact with him.

For the second part of this dare, you are going to connect with your man socially. Surprise him with a text message at work, simply telling him that you love him. Write him a love letter in his lunch box. If he wakes up before you for work, rise with him and pour his coffee. Remember your thankfulness part of your journal? You should be listing things about your husband you are thankful for. Perhaps you might include a few of these reasons in your love letter. Maybe you will plan something wonderful for the two of you, like an overnight stay at a Bed and Breakfast just outside your town, or a concert he would enjoy, or a dinner at a restaurant that is in your budget. Maybe, in your love letter, you can tell him that you want to reserve time this week to rent a movie, pop some popcorn, and curl up in front of the t.v. together. Choose a movie that you both will enjoy, one that doesn't include pregnancy or infant loss in its story line.

What are you sharing with your husband? Have you told him anything about your grief pregnancy activities at all? You might consider including in your love letter, what your feelings have been like, how you believe grief has challenged you, but how, through giving it nurturing, and giving it discipline, you are growing it into healing. Thank him for his patience and his grace as you explore the space that is grief.

Journal your plans, your fears and your hopes with this dare. When you have completed this week's challenges, write about your experiences in keeping a daily reminder to reach out and physically and socially connect with others – especially your spouse.

When You are Finished

Take time to congratulate yourself on revisiting these feelings.

Treat yourself to something relaxing or enjoyable.

I reflect in adoration on the gifts

my man has given me.

I determine to be fully present for him.

Your Sacred Space

__ DARE 20

This week, let's pause to see how far we've come.

In this middle place, I take respite.

You are neither in the newness of grief, nor have you quite yet met healing. In dare 18, we took some time to just be still with our grief, to allow ourselves to become more intimate and familiar with it. This week is a little different, in that we are going to look within and at ourselves, to see who we are as women, as mothers pregnant with grief.

My grief pregnancy tempts me to take shortcuts at almost every turn. The thoughts I allow to enter my mind are sometimes negative, selfish ones. I too often ignore my Self and indulge in the immaturity of my self. My mind feels distracted, hazy, heavy and forgetful.

I remember the challenge I gave myself to eat more nutritiously. I am honest in this time alone with my Self as I examine my diet. I have forsaken nutritious options for empty ones. I have been given opportunities to discipline my grief by giving living water to others, but I have complained at these opportunities and yet bemoaned my resulting condition of dryness.

The more people around me, the more alone I feel. I feel a disconnect, because I have allowed my self to silence my Self to such a quiet octave that I can't hear myself think. My short temper tells me what I somehow already know: there is clutter in my soul.

In truth, I didn't schedule these setbacks into my life. I charted on the calendar when I thought I'd be done with this grief pregnancy, and settled into the assumption that it would simply be so. I've allowed time to drag me into each day, achy and sore, with things left unnurtured and undisciplined from the day before pushing right along into this day with me.

I need this time. I need this space. I need to have an honest look at my self, and allow my Self to speak to me. In my quiet reflection, I am humbled to discover that, even though I have neglected my Self so poorly, my Self is still here. Still speaks ancient wisdom and profound truths to me.

I give myself time to be still. I hear the distractions my self fills me with, to turn me away from this sacred space. I allow each excuse and distraction to fade away. A spark of excitement stirs within me as I remember how fresh I came away from my last encounter with my Self. Like the phantom kicks of a pregnancy ended, something deep within me still remembers.

Revelations enter my soul through this time. I call into my mind the times I have cheated myself. The times I had that I neglected to nurture or to discipline my grief. I release emotions over this time of study. I evaluate these situations only with an eye on what I can take away, what I can carry, what I can bring into the next situation like it. Like a pregnant mother experiencing the first Braxton Hicks contractions, I practice in my mind's eye what living water I carry into the next squeeze.

What is nurturing my grief? Things that nurture my grief

speak love to me, validate the experiences I am having, give me the space I need to explore and grow.

What is disciplining my grief? There are many things, but mostly these are opportunities I am given that allow me to show myself that my grief really is growing in the direction of meeting my healing. When a baby is born, it is very common for the baby's head to begin to emerge, then slide back into the dark between the folds of the mother's secret place, to emerge again, and to repeat this process. Sliding backward is something that I didn't account for as I first plotted out what I thought my grief would be like, but is something that has value, when in proportion to the continued moving forward.

Things that discipline my grief are things that challenge me. They are encounters with everyday people and situations that result in my self having an encounter with my Self. The biggest version of me invites me to grow, to leave my pail. Things that discipline me begin by making me feel uncomfortable, and if I ignore the opportunity, I hush the voice of my Self a little more.

Preparing for labor is a kind of labor. If the selfish thoughts from my self are not quieted, they quickly grow so loud I spend my time pressing my hands over my ears in agony instead of allowing my hands to explore the space I am in and discover that I am on sacred ground.

Being still and being fully present in my time alone with my Self not only allows my grief pregnancy the discipline it needs, but it also allows for the nurturing that I so desperately crave.

I am called to times when my reaction was appropriate. I observe in my mind's eye as my Self leads me to a contraction that I endured in a very productive way. I faced the squeeze of an obstacle, a criticism, a challenge, and I used my techniques – breathing, Progressive Muscle Relaxation, healthy eating, positive reflection – the things I have come to know really only through this grief pregnancy.

As I feel this encounter ending, I am called to journal on these things, on these positive examples of my applications, on the growth I have identified in myself, and of the tools I have sharpened to make even more growth in the future.

Name the growth.

Preparation

Choose a private place where you feel comfortable and will have no interruptions (turn off your phone, and let others know not to disturb you).

Set aside enough time to do the activity so you do not feel rushed.

Plan to do something relaxing or enjoyable after you have finished the activity.

Try to relax (slow breathing) and clear your mind of other concerns before starting the activity.

The Dare

This was the dare just a couple of weeks ago: "Contemplate where you believe your grief may be leading you, what it may be preparing you for. Your grief should be leading you into a place that is new and that can seem scary, but a place that reveals the biggest version of your Self." This week, we are going to contemplate not on our grief, but on ourselves in our grief.

Evaluate honestly the quality of nurturing you have given your grief.

Evaluate honestly the quality of discipline you have given your grief.

You can type or handwrite, depending on your preference.

Do not be concerned with spelling, grammar, or punctuation.

Write your account in the first person (use "I" statements).

Write your account in the present tense (as if it is happening right now).

Include as much sensory detail as possible (sights, sounds, smells, textures, etc.)

Include any thoughts and feelings you had at the time.

Even though it may be painful, do not stop yourself from feeling emotions.

Keep writing until your account is complete, even if this takes a while.

When You are Finished

Take time to congratulate yourself on revisiting these feelings.

Treat yourself to something relaxing or enjoyable.

My grief pregnancy is being identified,

nurtured,

and disciplined.

My Sacred Space

Heidi Faith

__ DARE 21

This week, you and I, pregnant together in our grief journeys, are going to talk about menstruation.

What do birds and bees have to do with it?

Girlfriend, let's talk about it together. Get a warm cup of soothing broth – maybe it's tea, or cocoa, or coffee. One of my favorite drinks is a cup of fresh, frothy cocoa with a scoop of ice cold frozen homemade ice cream on top. Before it totally melts into the warmth, I sip, and my mouth collects a tiny morsel of cold cream in with the hot, sweet splash. My palate simply delights at the mix of extreme temperatures felt at the same time on my tongue.

The return of my menstrual cycle, and its candid calculation, was something I did not accept well. The reappearance of crimson, the color of my broken heart, felt to me as if my body had turned against me. Couldn't it hear the desires of my heart? My longing to have my baby once again? This, this mess I was faced with, seemed like a cruel joke. Even my body didn't listen to my plea. I felt abandoned even by my self.

The cramping of my uterus reminds me of an old, wrinkled

woman standing on a worn, wooden porch in front of a cabin in some remote place in the wilderness. She grasps firmly to a treasured, handmade quilt, a family heirloom handed down through the generations. She opens it to the wind, and with a firm grasp and steady thrust, dust flies off of this warm, worn blanket and scatter across the earth. In this way, this old woman is preparing to freshen the blanket for another use.

My uterus sheds and this wrinkled, old blanket somehow becomes refreshed, ready for life to enjoy its warmth. Even if no company comes and the blanket remains folded, perched on the armrest of the rocking chair, it is ready, and it is still a site to behold.

In my grief pregnancy, I fell out of love with my uterus.

Resentment fell upon me where marveling once captured my thoughts of it.

The whip of contractions felt constricted by my anxiety and anger. The pain magnified upon itself as my mind fed my soul junk – thoughts that could not possibly nourish.

I closed off when I needed to grow, to expand, to open, to release.

There are several scientific studies that indicate that when a mother is pregnant with a child, microscopic fragments of cells that belong to the child remain within the woman, forever. Physically, my body holds my child, forever.

Science confirms my invisible pregnancy.

For several weeks, this profound truth became my mantra. It beckons me to reflect on Mother Earth holding my baby in her womb, and on his physical form nourishing life.

What remains of him in me should also nourish life, but it is my job, my labor, to intentionally make this so.

I anticipate my next menstrual cycle. I prepare for the contractions, the physical cleansing of this priceless quilt, and I prepare for the emotional squeezes I know I will need to breathe and open myself to.

My body is not subject to my whims. It is not bound by the junk my self feeds me. I am overcome by the passionate persistence of my Self once again, for being my faithful friend no matter how I have silenced and ignored. My Self still speaks, still feeds, still loves me.

It took me several cycles to treasure this heirloom blanket. There are things that you might try as you spend time in that rocking chair, holding that quilt, tracing your fingers over its intricate stitching, whether you are hoping for company, hoping for some new person to borrow inside of it and be comforted by its warmth, or not.

Indulge in an intimate steam.

One such approach to admiring your wrinkled heirloom is the vaginal steam. It is a spa treatment that includes the steam of Mugwort and Wormwood. Mugwort is used in a technique called Moxibustion to help turn a breech baby to prepare him for birth. It is said to focus on stagnation and to encourage movement – the airing out of your quilt. Wormwood can be neurotoxic so it may or not be included in the vaginal steam, but its benefit is said to bring comfort to the pains of contractions – during birth or during menstruation.

Your delicate membranes may delight in this intentionally loving act. If, however, you simply don't feel this is for you, rest assured there are other ways to embrace all of the contractions that menstruation brings.

I need a hug, so I give myself one.

One of my most favorite things to do when my inner grandmother begins to air out her beautiful quilt is to hold something that reminds me of it. I purchased a rebozo, which is a thin, wide and long cotton scarf, and I wrap it around myself. Something about my womb can feel weak and unstable during menstruation. Wrapping a rebozo around myself feels safe. It allows me to be just as open as I need to be, without feeling as if this precious blanket is just going to fall out of my hands. Seeing myself in the mirror with this beautiful material embracing me reminds me that the desire to actually wrap myself came from my Self. I feel the squeezes of contractions. I feel the squeeze of my rebozo hold me through it all. I smile.

I have found a way to embrace the flow.

Preparation

Choose a private place where you feel comfortable and will have no interruptions (turn off your phone, and let others know not to disturb you).

Set aside enough time to do the activity so you do not feel rushed.

Plan to do something relaxing or enjoyable after you have finished the activity.

Try to relax (slow breathing) and clear your mind of other concerns before starting the activity.

The Dare

Spend time journaling about your body, about your menstruation, and about the messages you have been feeding your soul regarding menstruation and about the physical changes taking place in your body during your grief pregnancy.

You can type or handwrite, depending on your preference.

Do not be concerned with spelling, grammar, or punctuation.

Write your account in the first person (use "I" statements).

Write your account in the present tense (as if it is happening *right now*).

Include as much sensory detail as possible (sights, sounds, smells, textures, etc.)

Include any thoughts and feelings you had at the time.

Even though it may be painful, do not stop yourself from feeling emotions.

Keep writing until your account is complete, even if this takes a while.

When You are Finished

Take time to congratulate yourself on revisiting these feelings.

Treat yourself to something relaxing or enjoyable.

I carry living water.

My Sacred Space

Heidi Faith

___ DARE 22

This week, I am daring you to allow yourself to be seen by professionals.

I'm calling in the experts.

When is the last time you had a physical examination by a doctor? Have you yet had your follow-up appointment by an obstetrician or midwife after your pregnancy loss?

Preparation

Spend time carefully and honestly examining the needs of your physical body, listening to the messages your joints, your muscles, your bones send you. Is the pulse of your heart a joyful, enriching gushing into your vessel, or does it become too often dammed by anger, resentment and unhealth?

The birth of healing is something that takes a great deal of surrender. It takes nurturing grief and disciplining grief. It takes time. It takes solitude. In some ways, it also takes community. Allowing others to gather around you and give you the tools they have can grow your discernment on which of these tools is not needed, which may provide benefit, and which tools really are essential to the process. Remember, every mother's grief pregnancy is different.

The Dare

Purchase a new toothbrush. Consider scheduling an appointment with a chiropractor. Consider seeing your regular care provider. Perform regular breast examinations. Your vessel is magnificently interconnected and is majestically designed. Treat it with reverence.

This week, in addition to taking a practical look at these things, I want you to spend your early morning reflection time (if you are still doing this, fantastic! If you aren't, take a look back at dare nine. This is a dare that I encourage you to allow to become integrated into your life.) focusing on the images you have of your body.

Choose a private place where you feel comfortable and will have no interruptions (turn off your phone, and let others know not to disturb you).

Set aside enough time to do the activity so you do not feel rushed.

As you enter into this sacred space, allow your body to speak the messages you hear in your soul about this vessel you wear. Dance, sway, flow, rock, extend your arms and move your legs to the rhythm of the messages. When negative messages from your self enter, see them, and move them away. Talk out loud if you feel led to. Sing a beautiful hymn of enchantment and surrender to growth. When you are finished and believe you have exhausted this expression, spend time in a comfortable position, resting in the stillness.

Look into your special book or other place for your mantra. See if it relates to this exploration of your body.

As I complete this exercise, I am drawn once again to the woman at the well. I decide that I want to carry that picture with me throughout my day. I purchase a water bottle, one that is transparent so I can see the straw reaching deep into the bottom of the bottle. I carry this, my symbolic well, with me wherever I go. I am presented with one of my contractions – an encounter with an opportunity to discipline my grief – and I draw from my well. It quenches me, and I smile.

Spend time journaling about your body.

You can type or handwrite, depending on your preference.

Do not be concerned with spelling, grammar, or punctuation.

Write your account in the first person (use "I" statements).

Write your account in the present tense (as if it is happening right now).

Include as much sensory detail as possible (sights, sounds, smells, textures, etc.)

Include any thoughts and feelings you had at the time.

Even though it may be painful, do not stop yourself from feeling emotions.

Keep writing until your account is complete, even if this takes a while.

There can be freedom in asking for help.

When You are Finished

Take time to congratulate yourself on revisiting these feelings.

Treat yourself to something relaxing or enjoyable.

Heidi Faith

My water bottle quenches me in my grief pregnancy.

Heidi Faith

My water bottle quenches me in my grief pregnancy.

168

My Sacred Space

Heidi Faith

__ DARE 23

I often vacillate between believing I am either one extreme or another. This week's dare is to look at the impressions we have of ourselves, and the messages they speak to us.

I am little, but I am great.

Preparation

Spend time carefully and honestly examining the messages you send to your soul throughout the day. Empty messages of defeat don't simply wander into our minds and float into nothingness. They linger, and unless we sweep them out, we can quickly become consumed in junk.

The Dare

Purchase a small, glass jar, or use a small bowl. I decided on a flower pot, as I intend on this jar to grow something that lives long beyond the summer months of daisies. You may decide to decorate your jar with paint or inscribe special healing words and messages on it. Place it in a lovely spot in your home, such as a windowsill. Cut small scraps of colorful paper and place them in a container near the jar.

Now, consider the contractions as you labor into healing. There have already been so many contractions, cramps, situations where you felt your soul was squeezed. Situations where you didn't have all of the answers, but you did find a morsel. You found one, simple, treasured tool. Maybe it was deep, cleansing breathing. Perhaps it was holding your thoughts captive. Whatever it was, begin to jot down little notes, capturing these moments that you can find gratitude in.

I scribble little love notes to my Self.

From time to time, when you are enjoying your sacred space, pour these notes out around you, and read them. Journal your feelings on this.

Choose a private place where you feel comfortable and will have no interruptions (turn off your phone, and let others know not to disturb you).

Set aside enough time to do the activity so you do not feel rushed.

As you enter into this sacred space, allow your body to speak the messages you hear in your soul about your little greatness. Do these messages confirm or try to deny this truth? Dance, sway, flow, rock, extend your arms and move your legs to the rhythm of the messages. When negative messages from your self enter, see them, and move them away. Talk out loud if you feel led to. Sing a beautiful hymn of enchantment and surrender to growth. When you are finished and believe you have exhausted this expression, spend time in a comfortable position, resting in the stillness.

Lay down, with your spine aligned and your body relaxed. Sprinkle your love notes onto yourself. Guide your mind into exploring the liberating magnificence of your little greatness.

Spend time journaling about your little greatness.

You can type or handwrite, depending on your preference.

Do not be concerned with spelling, grammar, or punctuation.

Write your account in the first person (use "I" statements).

Write your account in the present tense (as if it is happening *right now*).

Include as much sensory detail as possible (sights, sounds, smells, textures, etc.)

Include any thoughts and feelings you had at the time.

Even though it may be painful, do not stop yourself from feeling emotions.

Keep writing until your account is complete, even if this takes a while.

When You are Finished

Take time to congratulate yourself on revisiting these feelings.

Treat yourself to something relaxing or enjoyable.

I am little, and I am great.

Heidi Faith

Your Sacred Space

__ DARE 24

This week, we are going to make bread together.

I will feed it and provide it with warmth.

When someone says, "I've got a bun in the oven" I always, immediately see Shadrach, Meshach, and Abednego in the roaring flames of a furnace.

"Gold is tested by fire, and human character is tested in the furnace of humiliation" – Sirach 2:5

What are your first thoughts when you see the word "humiliation"? I think of a flushed, red face, hot with embarrassment and maybe even a degree of shame, mixed in with some anger.

The thing is, I want my human character to grow. I know that someday, my physical form will feed the earth, and I want it to bring nourishment, not fill life with empty junk. My indwelled Self longs to be the well I can be, bringing living waters to those who thirst.

I need to see humiliation differently.

The root of humiliation is humble. As Charlotte, ever the faithful friend, explains to Wilbur the simple but profound word woven into her web in the classic book "Charlotte's Web", there is much more to this adjective.

Humiliation is the opposite of boastful. When one is boastful, they are "puffed up" with their own hot air. Being humble is to show submissive respect.

The way to submissive respect is through an honest assessment of your potential. And, there is only one way to obtain this honest assessment. It is to be fully present with your Self, presenting all of yourself to your Self, quieting your disruptive and intrusive thoughts of excuses and distractions, and allow your Self to draw back the thick curtains of habits, lies, selfishness, pride and shame.

Getting into a place where you can take down your defenses and open yourself up to a spiritual examination takes bravery, commitment and love. When you have reached this place where you can surrender your bucket to become a well, you will know that this place is most sacred, indeed.

In fact, the people of my most favorite book marked these special encounters by placing stones there, so that people after them who encounter these stones will know that flesh met Self and that these passersby are beholden to a sacred ground.

"Gold and silver are tested by fire, and a person's heart is tested by the Lord."
— Proverbs 17:3

When two Bible verses are so aligned in this way, it means that one is explaining the other. Meeting my Lord is to meet with my own humiliation. It is to face the things that would make our cheeks red, hot with embarrassment and anger, and it replaces these things we have allowed to grow that do not fuel the biggest life within us. The Gardener of my soul removes the false coverings of pride and shame from me and while I feel so often that my landscape is left a little too barren, a little too exposed and I am left a little too flat and empty by His tilling and toiling,

He waters that which will grow more abundantly through the agrology. More than that, He teaches me how, and He fills me with a well for which I can share this water with others.

How often I flee from the warmth of my furnace. My self lies to me, telling me to fear the furnace. The furnace brings life, it grows my Self. When the hot is just right, I will be refreshed by living water.

I marvel at Shadrach, Meshach, and Abednego for emerging from the furnace. I marvel at the woman who left her pail with Jesus. I marvel, because they each met their humiliation, their flattening, their emptying, but they grew from it. They didn't even boast in their true greatness – they immediately set out to share it, instead. I am little, and I am great.

My furnace still waits for me to still myself and let it warm me.

My furnace can nourish me,
just as my well can quench me.

We are going to begin a homemade sourdough starter together. You are going to feed your starter every day, and when it has been nurtured to the right growth, you will discipline it by the warmth of your oven. It will rise, and it will nourish.

My furnace holds eternal life.

Preparation

Gather the supplies needed to begin your sourdough starter.

The Dare

Each day, feed your sourdough starter. Enter into your sacred space and journal on the thoughts and feelings you have from the experience.

Homemade Sourdough Starter

Supplies:
Glass containers (at least two, Mason jars work well)
Towel to cover top
2-6 cups of flour, preferably sprouted or rye (directions for sprouted flour below)
2-6 cups filtered water

Directions:
Mix together 1 cup of the flour and 1 cup of the water in a glass container. Loosely cover the container with a towel (and rubber band if necessary). Allow to sit in a warm spot in your kitchen where it won't be disturbed.

Each day, for up to a week, transfer your mixture to a new, clean bowl with a new addition of ½ cup water and ½ cup flour. After a few days, you will notice the starter will become slightly bubbly and develop a "wine-like" aroma.

Your starter will be ready to bake in a recipe of your choosing after this week.

Continue to feed your starter with equal parts sprouted flour and filtered water in a fresh jar every day.

Your starter can live this way
for many, many years.

The directions for sprouted flour are located here: *modernnourishment.wordpress.com/2012/12/05/how-we-make-our-sprouted-flour/*

To find this starter recipe on the web, please visit *modernnourishment.wordpress.com*

I think of Jesus feeding what seemed like the whole world, with only a couple of fish and a few meager loaves of bread. Is the little loaf of my Self that has been nurtured by living water and disciplined in the furnace of my Self really enough to feed, to satisfy the spiritual hunger of my community, my world? This book, The Invisible Pregnancy, is a crumb I offer to you to taste. It's just a crumb. I give it to you, hoping it will nourish you. Somehow, I am not left empty by the sharing, but instead it grows me in some mysterious, rich way.

This week, as you feed your sourdough starter, journal your thoughts on the experience.

You can type or handwrite, depending on your preference.

Do not be concerned with spelling, grammar, or punctuation.

Write your account in the first person (use "I" statements).

Write your account in the present tense (as if it is happening right now).

Include as much sensory detail as possible (sights, sounds, smells, textures, etc.)

Include any thoughts and feelings you had at the time.

Even though it may be painful, do not stop yourself from feeling emotions.

Keep writing until your account is complete, even if this takes a while.

When You are Finished

Take time to congratulate yourself on revisiting these feelings.

Treat yourself to something relaxing or enjoyable.

Your Sacred Space

__ DARE 25

Now that our bread is ready for baking, let's prepare a special meal and dine together.

We let our sacraments nourish us.

If feeding and growing a living bread brought nourishment to you, warming it in your oven and pairing it with a special beverage will be a very lovely treat. If you haven't begun to grow your living bread, or if your process is taking a few tries, that is just fine. You can wait on this dare, or you can purchase a loaf of fresh baked Challah or French bread from your local bakery.

For this dare, I invite you to partake of one of my favorite drinks. Paired with your living bread, this will make a wonderful evening snack that should be had during time in your sacred space. If you decide to make a supper with these items, I recommend bringing in your favorite recipe of prepared fresh fish.

How is your twelfth dare coming along? The dare that introduced the idea of eating foods that are fresh and served in their most natural state. Have you yet prepared a banquet for your beloved? This week's dare may inspire you to complete that dare, or, to revisit it and do it again!

One of my most favorite drinks is a bouquet of freshly picked fruit, mingled beautifully with the deep, dry bitterness of red wine, which is overcome by the life of carbonated water.

Known as *Sangria*, this is a complex blend of flavors and feelings, that is easy to make.

You might mix freshly squeezed lemonade or orange juice into your batch, splash in some ginger ale and the wine of your selection, and toss in slices of fresh strawberries, oranges, limes, or sprinkle in some cherries. Use your imagination and resourcefulness in whatever season finds you in taking on this dare.

If an event or person (including your Self) has ever indicated that consuming alcohol, even in moderation, is an unwise decision for you to make, if you are under the legal drinking age, or if you simply prefer, you can substitute sparkling juice for the wine.

Only one more item is needed, and you will be ready for your time in your sacred space. Gather the items: your bread (uncut), your sangria, and include a candle.

Perhaps you will sit at your dining room table, or you may find you desire to pack an outdoor picnic or, you may decide to hold an indoor picnic sitting comfortably on the floor.

There are so many opportunities to revisit previous dares and bring this into them. Where did you go for dare eleven, when you became fully present in the outdoors?

Wherever this dare invites you to enjoy your living sacraments, get comfortable in your space, and light your candle.

I invite you to become fully present during this time. Reflect on dare twelve where getting present while eating was first introduced.

In your space, contemplate that which you know about the

value of the furnace. The warmth of your baby's physical transformation is nourishing the earth. The warmth of your oven grew your living bread and prepared it for your consumption. The warmth that is your Self is a fire within you.

When you and your husband married, did you each take a lit candle and join them into a third candle? I enjoy this imagery and find great value in it.

In my sacred space, I breathe in, deeply.

I exhale fear and tension.

I breathe in, again, more deeply than before. I feel the oxygen moving through my body.

I again, exhale, feeling more refreshed and more relaxed.

I study the spread that lay before me. I hold my glass of Sangria up to my nose and breathe in the beautiful, exotic, deep and fresh smells. My mouth waters. I take a sip.

My hands find the bread and hold it reverently. My fingers feel the smooth coarseness of the shell. Pushing deep, my hands break through the crust into the soft, pillowy center. Crumbs fall and spread.

I look at my candle. I study the flame. I hold the bread that was made into something that can nourish me because of the blaze of the furnace.

This moment is so powerful, so sacred, I am moved to tears.

My self rushes in with lies, telling me that I am weeping over what was lost, that these are tears of anger and that my anger is justified, that my feelings of despair should be fed, that I should allow my longings to grow.

Oh, but I have already come to the well. I have already sat near the furnace and felt its power. My Self has grown within me, I am growing into healing. I know these tears are my surrender, my allowing my well to grow deeper, my allowing my Gardener to till the soil even when I think that I am still too fragile, too bruised, too exposed from His work.

I become open in a way
that I haven't known.

I weep, and words declaring my total adoration for the selfless Self escape breathily and easily from my lips. I profess my reverence for the mysterious power that isn't me yet indwells deep within my well. My Self is growing, fed from simple crumbs of humility and small sips of living water. I am nurturing and disciplining my grief pregnancy and a presence is becoming so noticeable within me that my skin glows radiantly and I feel a life force stirring within.

I chew and sip in silence,
keenly aware that I am not alone.

Preparation

Gather the supplies needed to make your Sangria, and gather your beautiful drink, your fresh bread, and your candle, and create a sacred space for your meal.

The Dare

Bake your sourdough starter by your favorite recipe's instructions. Pair it with homemade Sangria, and if you'd like, fresh fish to make a complete meal. Bring and light a candle. Enter fully into your sacred space with your meal and your Self.

When you have finished your meal, journal your thoughts on the experience.

You can type or handwrite, depending on your preference.

Do not be concerned with spelling, grammar, or punctuation.

Write your account in the first person (use "I" statements).

Write your account in the present tense (as if it is happening right now).

Include as much sensory detail as possible (sights, sounds, smells, textures, etc.)

Include any thoughts and feelings you had at the time.

Even though it may be painful, do not stop yourself from feeling emotions.

Keep writing until your account is complete, even if this takes a while.

When You are Finished

Take time to congratulate yourself on revisiting these feelings.

Treat yourself to something relaxing or enjoyable.

Your Sacred Space

__ DARE 26

In dare twenty, we looked at the emotional aspects of being somewhere in the middle of our grief pregnancies. This week, we are going to examine the physical nature of finding ourselves somewhere in a strange middle place.

How do I care for my vessel?

As a mother's body changes to accommodate the growth of a child nestled within, she finds her form changing, expanding, and filling in ways that can be marvelous or can be frightening. After the birth of your baby, in any trimester, your body still may hold some of these changes. Some mothers cling to any resemblance of carrying their child, and they try to maintain this shape through consuming extra calories. Still other times, the grief pregnancy can seem to make carrying her own bucket such a wearisome burden that exercise seems daunting. And there are mothers yet who try to quickly rush themselves through their grief pregnancy so that they can become pregnant with a child again. Yes, it is possible to become pregnant with a child at any point in your grief pregnancy. You are wise to be gentle on yourself and care for your grief pregnancy; if you become pregnant with a child during this time, you will need to care for your growing child, and the most optimal way to do this is to already hold a presence in your grief pregnancy, giving it the nurturance and the discipline it needs.

So, how do we care for ourselves in this middle place? Maternity clothes may be too big. They also may be too big of a painful reminder. Your previous, non-maternity clothes, however, are too snug. Oh, how to usher in one or the other!

Be present in this middle place. Enter into it. Allow your Self to speak affirmations of your worth, your abilities, your beauty, your value in this middle place.

Your Self is growing, every day. Practice, in this middle place, being full of Self. Being full of Self means shedding the self, and the lies, shame and pride that it uses to try to fill you with junk.

I am.

You know you are becoming filled with Self when the messages you become filled with are "I am" messages. Practice some with me:

I am curious.

I am eating, chewing, tasting my food.

I am sitting through a very long meeting at work. I am chewing on my pen. I am not feeling very present through this lecture.

I am hungry.

I am entering into my sacred space.

This moment is your life. Be present in it. Allow it to manifest to its greatest potential.

Take an honest assessment of your appearance, including your wardrobe. Does it reflect your being fully present in your middle place, or does it indicate a wistfulness or a distraction from where you currently are?

Preparation

Take an honest look at your wardrobe. Does it reveal any cloaking or shrouding in mistruths or distractions, or do your clothes fit you well? If you need to, begin to budget in a little indulgence. This week, I'd like you to go to Victoria Secret's or other professional lingerie boutique, and get professionally fitted for a properly sized bra.

The Dare

Begin to budget in for the purchase of a nice, new bra. There is such a beautifully feminine feeling in allowing a professional, a woman, to wrap her measuring tape around your bosom and guide you in finding the dimensions of one of the most womanly parts of your body.

Depending on your finances, get professionally sized for free, and then visit a larger chain retailer to purchase a new bra (Kmart, Walmart or other places have beautiful bras).

When you have finished this dare, journal your thoughts on the experience. What was it like, during your outing? Did you or do you plan on telling your man about it? Did you make a purchase? Did you hear any messages from your self, whispering lies of inferiority, wistfulness or shame? Did you allow your Self to move these messages away and replace them with fully present, I am, messages?

You can type or handwrite, depending on your preference.

Do not be concerned with spelling, grammar, or punctuation.

Write your account in the first person (use "I" statements).

Write your account in the present tense (as if it is happening right now).

Include as much sensory detail as possible (sights, sounds, smells, textures, etc.)

Include any thoughts and feelings you had at the time.

Even though it may be painful, do not stop yourself from feeling emotions.

Keep writing until your account is complete, even if this takes a while.

When You are Finished

Take time to congratulate yourself on revisiting these feelings.

Treat yourself to something relaxing or enjoyable.

Your Sacred Space

Heidi Faith

__ DARE 27

We've talked about situations in which a baby's physical form is buried. We've talked about when a baby's physical form enters into the waterways, either through a trail of life beginning with burial, or when a baby's physical form is flushed. These are difficult things to talk about. This week, we are going to talk about when a baby's physical form is cremated.

Beauty from ashes...

Sometimes a hospital will offer to cremate the physical form of the baby collectively; more than one physical forms are gathered together – perhaps they all had been born via miscarriage, or perhaps one or more of these babies had been born via elective abortion for any of a number of reasons. For financial, practical, or policy reasons, this group cremation may be performed.

Still other parents gather the physical form of their baby, and/or placenta, and bring it to a crematorium to have it cremated.

After the baby's physical form is cremated, a cemetery may

hold the baby's name on a special plaque, the family may then bury the ashes, scatter them, or may place all or some of them in a special vase or jewelry piece made for this purpose.

For this week, we are going to focus on an activity that gives intentional love to these parents. We are going to engage in an activity that involves a dry, dusty powder, similar to dust.

From dust to dust…

Preparation

A 3 ft. x 4 ft. chalkboard and some colorful chalk would work very well, but any sized chalkboard will do. For a more ongoing version of this dare, consider purchasing some chalkboard paint, and reserve a special section of wall, perhaps in the room where you find your sacred space waiting for you.

Additional items for an activity that is an extension of the first one include gathering plenty of old magazines, including any parenting magazines that you may have registered for during your time in pregnancy with your child. A large posterboard, scissors, glue or tape, and maybe even a picture frame will be needed. You can shop at a thrift store to select an old print and remove the frame.

The Dare

Begin by entering into your sacred space, with your supplies.

Call into your mind the messages that your Self gifts you with, that give you impressions of what your life will look like when you meet your healing.
What will your life be like? What will you be like, when you give birth to healing?

As these messages come to you, write them on your chalkboard. Write them in different colors if you choose. Allow your Self to create a beautiful mosaic of affirmations for you to gaze at and meditate on.

I will share with you some of the words that my Self revealed to me during my time examining these messages and images. I allowed my Self to speak these messages to me in the *I am*.

I am wise.

I am empathetic.

I am a deep well of living water.

I am a vessel that holds life bigger than me.

I am a mother.

I am a bereaved mother, who has experienced being pregnant with grief.

I am a bereaved mother, who has shaped my grief into healing.

I am a mother, who has learned that being in healing is a different kind of being in grief.

I am aware that my grief hasn't simply vanished into nothingness, but that it has transformed.

I am aware that my child hasn't simply vanished into nothingness, but that my child's physical form has transformed.

I am aware that my child hasn't simply vanished into nothingness, but that my child's spiritual form has transformed.

I am growing.

I am able to have setbacks.

I am able to identify my strengths.

I am capturing my thoughts.

I am surrendering to my Self.

I am healing.

I am.

I filled my chalkboard faster than I thought I would. I marvel at the frenzy with which the words came flowing out. I study the chalk on my hands. I gaze intently at the colorful dust that sprinkled onto my carpet, my clothes, and that pushed into the lines and wrinkles of my fingertips. I decide firmly that indeed, dust can bring healing.

I keep my smudging of affirmations. I dwell on them, and allow them to become my mantras.

On another day during the week, again, enter into your sacred space holding the thought of beauty from ashes. Look through your large stack of old magazines. Seek images that reflect the feelings that are invoked when you speak your dusty mosaic of mantras. Is there a woman, glowing and smiling? Does she look refreshed? Rip or cut it out, and paste it to your posterboard. Fill this space with images, hidden in places that may otherwise be considered rubbish. These images feed your Self and reveal the experience you are growing toward, preparing to meet your healing. After your posterboard is completely filled, add on to the concept of beauty from ashes by purchasing an old, framed piece of art from your local thrift store, and use it's frame to hold your colorful art. You can do this by carefully removing the paper under the glass, or simply by taping your piece on top of the glass. Dwell on your mosaic of messages.

When you are done with these activities, journal on your experiences.

You can type or handwrite, depending on your preference.

Do not be concerned with spelling, grammar, or punctuation.

Write your account in the first person (use "I" statements).

Write your account in the present tense (as if it is happening right now).

Include as much sensory detail as possible (sights, sounds, smells, textures, etc.)

Include any thoughts and feelings you had at the time.

Even though it may be painful, do not stop yourself from feeling emotions.

Keep writing until your account is complete, even if this takes a while.

When You are Finished

Take time to congratulate yourself on revisiting these feelings.

Treat yourself to something relaxing or enjoyable.

Name your pieces. There is a special power in claiming these pieces as yours, and of gifting your work with a name. Snap a photo of each piece to include in your journal.

Your Sacred Space

__ DARE 28

In dare twenty-three, we looked at the impressions we have of ourselves. We began to write little love notes to our Selves. How is that going for you? How many times have you filled your jar with wonderful observations of your little greatness?

I am little, but I am great.

We are building a depth, a height, and a presence that we didn't know existed before. We are growing a living entity within us. We are nurturing and disciplining our grief pregnancy to allow our Selves the most optimum room for growth as we prepare to meet our healing.

This week, I want to meet you in your sacred space. I want to sit Burmese next to you. I want to wrap my hands around a warm cup of love steeped in comfort, and I want us to share some of the most philosophically profound thoughts in a gentle and easy way together, you and I, we two mothers.

During a grief pregnancy, many a mother will set out on two different but important missions: one, to identify the physical reasons for the loss of her child, and two, to understand the spiritual reasons for the loss of her child.

My precious, courageous friend, I place my hand gently atop yours, gaze into your beautiful eyes, as I whisper to you,

these pages hold neither answer.

When I search my soul regarding these things, and invite my Self to speak, this is what I hear:

Every loss happens for a physical reason, but even within that physical reason,
   there is a spiritual reason.

The spiritual reason is never to punish you, nor is it to punish your child.

I believe in the one God of the universe, the Great Gardener who toils over Mother Earth and who tills and fills my soul. Yet, even others who believe in this same God, believe different things than I do. Some believe that God is a helpless, heartbroken bystander that spun the little Dreidel called earth and who now only observes as it tips over. Still others believe that not only did God orchestrate the events that directly led to your pregnancy loss, but that God wanted your loss to occur.

My beliefs find their place somewhere in the middle of what I see as these two extremes.

I believe that once I surrendered my life, once I identified that there is a Great Gardener and that I can grow best by admitting that His view of my landscape is much larger, more complete and even more beautiful than I could ever see through my self, I quieted my frail, ineffective plow. I turned off the shrubbery shears which were too heavy for me to coordinate safely. I set down my leaking watering jar. I believe that once I did these things, I discovered for the first time a mysterious, magical seed embedded within my soul. I marveled that this seed had been there as far back as I was just a seed myself, but that I never even once thought to notice it before.
   The event that drew me to this surrender was when I became

pregnant for the first time, and felt the magnitude and enormity of motherhood. I was so overcome by the sense that God knew I would be a mother for the rest of my life, that I knew I would be a mother for the rest of my life! There was such a deep sense of expectation and stability that came with the discovery of my motherhood, I knew that I had not given myself this gift, but that it had been given to me by someone much more stable than my self.

Through that first pregnancy, I learned to feed and water this seed. As the seed grew, I knew what it was and what it was growing into. It was the seed of my Self, growing into the biggest version of me. This seed is a spirit; it is not mine but it indwells within me. It is a holy spirit, meaning, it is all good. It cannot do, provoke or become evil.

So, you see, my first pregnancy was a gift. It wasn't a gift of appreciation for my ignoring the squeaky whisper of the infinitesimal seed I had not recognized was in me. No, my first pregnancy wasn't a gift of approval. I was with a man who was dangerous and I haphazardly settled on filling my vessel with his junk and allowed myself to starve, spiritually. I did not deserve any applause for my spiritual laziness.

I was given the seed of this child, to help me identify the seed of my Self. The Great Gardener, in His infinite wisdom and view of my landscape, knew that implanting the one seed would give me the better view of the other. By learning to care for the one, I began to care for the other.

My Great Gardener is merciful. He wants the biggest, fullest, richest life in His garden. He allows me to help with my meager contribution, and He is tender in His discipline as I destroy some parts and as I leave other parts untended.

Since my first pregnancy, I have learned to care for this seed of Self, and have watched it grow and mature. The more I listen, the more clear it speaks to my soul, and the more I have learned to heed its word.

So, why, then, would any of the other seeds of life be removed from the soil of my womb? Why would I endure a pregnancy loss?

Was this somehow, punishment to me? Did I somehow owe my Great Gardener?

Was He somehow, foreclosing on and seizing the property of my landscape? Didn't I already give it to Him?

In the newness of my grief, I was angry at my Gardener. I thought about firing Him, or demoting Him, at least. And in some ways, in honest reflection, for a time I believe I did. I felt too vulnerable. I felt I had given Him too much control. I wanted to take it back. I wanted my pregnancy back.

Even when I discovered that I had a well within me, I was still discouraged. I wanted my little bucket back instead.

I can absolutely say that my first pregnancy was an undeserved gift. It was an invitation to see the seed of Self, and I took the invitation.

Is every pregnancy an undeserved gift?

What about mothers who become pregnant through enduring rape?

Is every pregnancy an undeserved gift?

Yes. I do believe that every pregnancy is an undeserved gift.

Even the pregnancy that did not bring forth the life that I anticipated, that I hoped for, that I assumed it would.

I am not ashamed to say that I flat assumed my pregnancy would bring forth a living baby, for me to nurture and raise.

Because, you see, friend, let me lean in even closer to tell you. Let me take my finger and gently tuck the wisp of your bangs from your face and secure it behind your lovely ear:

Your grief pregnancy is an undeserved gift.

I didn't deserve to lose my pregnancy, my child. I didn't deserve the sense of abandonment, cruelty and vulnerability, physically and spiritually, the experience subjected me to.

But through the darkness, through the storm, of these horrendous attacks, I found that my Self had deepened, had grown.

Your grief pregnancy is filled with wonder, with mystery, with magic. I don't know the physical or the spiritual reasons for your becoming pregnant with grief, but I can tell you that you are a treasure. Your landscape is stunning. It is marvelous to behold. Your Great Gardener looks lovingly upon you, and your landscape is fertile with life that is infinitely bigger than you can see with the eyes of your self.

In your grief pregnancy, as you identify, nurture and discipline your Self, you will give birth to healing. You will behold the life force that has been within you, is of you, but is not you. Even without all of the answers your heart yearns to know, you will find that you are in a space that is sacred, that your landscape is fertile, and that your garden is holy.

Somehow, the conversations in my heart that involve these things, that involve this tilling in my mind and this watering of my emotions, they manifest into the conversations around me. When I have allowed my self to grow the weeds of anger, accusation, and frustration, because I don't have or don't fully understand the physical or the spiritual reasons for my pregnancy loss, I find that I am much more curt to those around me. I become abrasive and cutting to them. I become distanced and distracted, as these weeds of insecurity block my vision and my connection. I need to discipline my Self, call it forward, become fully present in the moment I am in, and capture my thoughts.

What about you?

Do you have structured fences in how you argue? Do you argue well? Do you connect well? This week's dare is about looking at arguing well, and about connecting well.

Preparation

Choose a private place where you feel comfortable and will

have no interruptions (turn off your phone, and let others know not to disturb you).

Set aside enough time to do the activity so you do not feel rushed.

Plan to do something relaxing or enjoyable after you have finished the activity.

Try to relax (slow breathing) and clear your mind of other concerns before starting the activity.

Who are your girlfriends? Has this list changed since you became pregnant with grief? During this dare, you will plan an old fashioned slumber party. Invite and have confirmed at least two women who you enjoy being around. Whether at your home, a lodge, a Bed and Breakfast, or a hotel, plan on having an overnight together. The more extravagant your plans become, remember to accommodate your husband as well. This is a ladies evening, but he should feel comfortable in the planning too, so let him know that you intend on a ladies slumber party, and make arrangements that allow him a comfortable night as well.

Plan games, such as Twister, card games, or getting to know you games. Plan a pillow fight! Think on food, snacks and beverages to include. You might want to gift your friends with a batch of your living bread, or you might want to prepare a carafe of Sangria. Maybe you'll have a collection of love movies or silly comedies to watch. Consider asking each woman to bring something silly, or to be ready to chat about something that gives them great hope or satisfaction.

You don't have to plan your slumber party to commence by the end of the week. In fact, a great overnight will require planning, imagination and budgeting. This week, you will work on setting the first steps in motion to complete this dare. For you, that might mean making the first connections to build friendships. Maybe you know of someone who you can gift The Invisible Pregnancy book to, with a little note that bookmarks this dare, sending them a warm message that you are available when they reach this dare.

The Dare

Part one: meditate and journal on the ways that you argue, particularly with your spouse. Has the way you argue changed since becoming pregnant with grief? Call into your soul an action plan to argue well. Even if your spouse doesn't have his own action plan, determine to commit to yours. Explore ways in your sacred space how your Self can bring arguments into opportunities to connect and heal, rather than to cut and divide. You should still be adding to your thankfulness list, writing the things you are thankful for in your husband. As you hold this growing list, of the simple, of the daily, of the too often overlooked opportunities you've had to water his soul, allow your feelings to cry out in adoration of him. Beneath the weeds of his own anger and hurt, his Self longs to connect with yours. His Self doesn't want to hurt you. The next time your tempers meet each others, remember to allow the argument to become an undeserved gift.

Part two: prepare your slumber party with your girlfriends, and journal on the planning, and on the event.

When you are done with these activities, journal on your experiences.

You can type or handwrite, depending on your preference.

Do not be concerned with spelling, grammar, or punctuation.

Write your account in the first person (use "I" statements).

Write your account in the present tense (as if it is happening right now).

Include as much sensory detail as possible (sights, sounds, smells, textures, etc.)

Include any thoughts and feelings you had at the time.

Even though it may be painful, do not stop yourself from feeling emotions.

Keep writing until your account is complete, even if this takes a while.

When You are Finished

Take time to congratulate yourself on revisiting these feelings.

Treat yourself to something relaxing or enjoyable.

My Self is an undeserved gift.

Heidi Faith

My Sacred Space

__ DARE 29

In this dare, we are going to do some journaling. This is an extended writing project that will build upon itself through the week.

I am connecting through writing.

You are going to journal about a fictitious friend. You are going to conjure her up, this fictitious friend, and imagine that she too, has experienced pregnancy loss. I want you to imagine that this friend has shared with you all of her thoughts and feelings about her experience. Because she has shared these things with you, you know how the trauma of her experience has impacted her life, and you know the meaning she has placed on her experience.

Journal a little, about the situation and experience of this fictitious friend. Allow this part of the dare to extend into a couple of days' thinking, if needed.

As you finish your journaling, spend time to return to her

scenario and, empathize with her experience. Read her story slowly.

Reflect on any strong feelings she has (guilt, shame, anger). Underline what seem to be her "hot spots".

Make space in your journaling to challenge any unhelpful core beliefs and thinking styles she has, challenge any unhelpful behavior patterns she has, and consider any positive consequences of her experience that she may not be able to see.

In the final part of the dare, you are going to journal a letter to your fictitious friend, as if you were confiding in her, but keep this letter as part of your journal.

In your letter to her, summarize what has happened to you; what you have experienced.

Reflect on the therapeutic and spiritual process you have encountered.

Include your insights, helpful experiences, changes in thinking, feeling and behavior).

Describe your relationship now, to your grief, and to your experience (helpful strategies, helpful ways of thinking, feeling or behaving).

Preparation

Choose a private place where you feel comfortable and will have no interruptions (turn off your phone, and let others know not to disturb you).

Set aside enough time to do the activity so you do not feel rushed.

Plan to do something relaxing or enjoyable after you have finished the activity.

Try to relax (slow breathing) and clear your mind of other concerns before starting the activity.

The Dare

Part one: journal the experiences of a fictitious friend who endured pregnancy loss.

Part two: contemplate on her story and experience. As you spend time contemplating on her story, note any differences or similarities you allowed there to be to your own experience, and why this might be. Journal a letter to her.

You can type or handwrite, depending on your preference.

Do not be concerned with spelling, grammar, or punctuation.

Write your account in the first person (use "I" statements).

Write your account in the present tense (as if it is happening *right now*).

Include as much sensory detail as possible (sights, sounds, smells, textures, etc.)

Include any thoughts and feelings you had at the time.

Even though it may be painful, do not stop yourself from feeling emotions.

Keep writing until your account is complete, even if this takes a while.

When You are Finished

Take time to congratulate yourself on revisiting these feelings.

Treat yourself to something relaxing or enjoyable.

Even when I feel that I don't have all I want from my experience, I still find that I have something to give to another.

Your Sacred Space

Heidi Faith

___ DARE 30

This week, we are going to become aware of the cycles in our life.

I move to an ebb and a flow that
I am becoming aware of.

This is a great place to pause, once again, and really examine the work you've accomplished in your grief pregnancy.

How many dares have spoken a hidden message to you that I did not write? How many times did your Self reveal something to you, a treasure, which you only found by submitting to the process and work of your grief pregnancy?

Looking back, what dares have been your favorites? Why?

What dares have you started but not fully completed?

Have you included more raw and fresh foods into your diet? Had that dare prompted you to resume taking a multivitamin?

Are you continuing in the activity you determined was

enjoyable and practical to integrate into your life?

Are you filling up your journal with thankful observations of your husband?

Are you filling up your jar with love notes from your Self?

Have you been feeding your living bread each day?

Are you still rising a bit earlier in the day than you used to, to ensure you have time to be in your sacred space?

Have you regularly held your thoughts captive? Have you held your thoughts captive during particularly stressful times, such as in wistfulness in seeking answers to your pregnancy loss, or when facing certain people, events, or situations, such as during intercourse or when menstruation begins?

Within your own unique grief pregnancy, some of these activities will need to be repeated. They will need to be approached again. They will need to be applied again, and again. You will need to continue to dare yourself.

That's OK.

Making allowance for setbacks is good. As they occur, use them as opportunities to evaluate your approach, and to continue to make your goals smarter, when needed. Consider this:

Your goals should be:

Specific – avoid vague goals. Establish what you want to achieve, how you will do it, when you will do it, where you will do it, and how often you will do it. Beginning with time in your sacred space and journaling is very important.

Measurable – seek ways to measure your progress so that you can tell your self when your goal has been achieved. Go to your jar, watch it fill, to stay motivated.

Attainable – allow your Self to speak honestly to you, and be open to listening if your goal is truly realistic. Your goals should positively challenge you.

Rewarding – your goals should be rewarding and meaningful to you. When you are familiar with your reasons for wanting to attain a goal, it is more likely that achieving it will be rewarding to you.

Timely – being specific, but not rigid, with the timeframes in working toward you goal can help you reach it.

Evaluate – making allowances for setbacks in proportion to your growth is helpful. For example: "I will take a 10 minute walk, once every day." Speak an I am statement in your allowance, such as "I am choosing not to take my 10 minute walk today. I have accomplished my goal every day this week, and I am going to walk again tomorrow." Noting your accomplishments – identifying your little greatness – is important.

Review – as you move nearer to your goal, you may gain a better vision of any improvement or revision your goal may need. You will be able to review your skills and abilities, and determine what resources you may need in reaching your goal. Either you goal may need to be changed, or you may need more support in reaching it.

As you read through the way to SMARTER goals, enter into your sacred space and contemplate the goals you have in your life. Check them against this little checklist. Journal on what your Self speaks to you. Write down any new goals revealed to you in this sacred space.

As I anticipate giving birth to healing,
I begin to write my birth plan.

Preparation

Choose a private place where you feel comfortable and will have no interruptions (turn off your phone, and let others know not to disturb you).

Set aside enough time to do the activity so you do not feel rushed.

Plan to do something relaxing or enjoyable after you have finished the activity.

Try to relax (slow breathing) and clear your mind of other concerns before starting the activity.

The Dare

Journaling your goals as you prepare to meet your healing unfolds into writing your birth plan. In your sacred space, write the goals you have as your laboring opens you and brings you to meeting your healing. What aspects of this experience are within your control? Breathing, progressive muscle relaxation, a well fed and properly exercised body, a well fed and well watered soul, are all well within you to accomplish. What other aspects of your environment have you helped to shape? Have you invited into your space people who are trustworthy, people who have an intuitive love for you, people who validate your labor? Have you been merciful to forgive those parts of themselves that do not serve you to the fullest of your desires but to the fullest they are currently capable? Have you identified the needs that require support from experts, such as a dentist, physical therapist, a pastor, or a social worker? Your grief pregnancy is different than any other mothers, and yet it shares some foundational similarities to every mother ever pregnant with grief. Some contractions of offense you will handle gracefully and easily. Others will invoke you to pause and to rely on tools, teachings and practices that you'll need to have practiced – things you've learned in this guide. Some parts of your laboring will progress will require patience, and a trust in the moments in waiting, even if there are many. Some parts of your laboring will require your quieting your selfish self and will only be accomplished through connecting, through touching, through interacting, through permitting others into your sacred space.

Let your thoughts drift to your goals. Present them, one at a time, to your Self. Listen.

When you are finished contemplating on your goals and listening to your Self speak encouragement and guidance in relation to your goals, journal on your experience.

You can type or handwrite, depending on your preference.

Do not be concerned with spelling, grammar, or punctuation.

Write your account in the first person (use "I" statements).

Write your account in the present tense (as if it is happening right now).

Include as much sensory detail as possible (sights, sounds, smells, textures, etc.)

Include any thoughts and feelings you had at the time.

Even though it may be painful, do not stop yourself from feeling emotions.

Keep writing until your account is complete, even if this takes a while.

When You are Finished

Take time to congratulate yourself on revisiting these feelings.

Treat yourself to something relaxing or enjoyable.

Heidi Faith

Your Sacred Space

__ DARE 31

Just as a mother's growing belly when she is pregnant with a child invokes unsolicited advice and dramatic stories, your grief pregnancy has likely brought some unsolicited comments, unhelpful perspectives and unneeded comparisons or expectations of others.

You likely endured more of this than you could have possibly imagined in the earliest days of your grief pregnancy. The contractions of offense and hurt squeezed your soul, as this entity embedded deep within you began to take root. I bring these things up now, though, because as you near the first encounter with your healing, you will discover that there are new offenses: unsolicited expectations and comparisons of your laboring. As you continue to hold the thoughts of your manifesting birth plan, take time this week to identify the contractions that you feel now, that are new, but that hurt in a similar way to the hurts in your earliest days in this grief pregnancy.

In the later days of my grief pregnancy, I found that the tools I had in place to help me through my laboring were scrutinized by others. I discovered that someone stole the name of my website, and I had to make a legal plan and give a loving approach. Someone else had tried to steal a great portion of my writing. Still another person published bizarre untruths about me and my website. I was accused of being too Christian. I was accused of not being Christian enough.

I was hurt at these offenses, and sometimes allowed myself to believe that they were separate from my grief pregnancy, that they were each isolated offenses, and that I was isolated from others in these experiences. It took quiet time in my sacred space for my Self to speak to me, to comfort me, to reveal to me the profound truth that all bereaved mothers face these laboring pains. That they reach a point in their grief pregnancy where they are invited – where they are forced – to labor through the contractions with all of the techniques, with all of the skills, with all of the trusted fellowship, with all of the love, with all of the patience, with all of the help they can get.

When it feels as if you must surely be starting all the way over, when it feels as if you must surely not have grown at all, when it feels as if you must surely be failing, be still, precious friend. Enter into your sacred space. Listen to your Self speak. You are almost done.

I dwell on the mantra I have been given. Trust in the process. I feel "overdue" for healing. I feel annoyed with my circumstances and frustrated with others' thoughtlessness. I feel wounded and vulnerable.

I journal on criticism and on loneliness. The pain of disappointment squeezes and reminds me that others can't fill my water jar. Why do I keep turning to social media, to the words of strangers for approval? They give chaotic splashes of affection when my need is so much deeper. I become able to identify my begging for a scrap and can discipline this behavior.

I think on a woman I've read about. She bled for years. She bled so long and so much that she tried everything she could think of to try to get it to stop. She tried the traditional medicinal doctors of the time. She tried sorcery, which is to draw from the spiritual well while ignoring the presence of the Gardener who beckons to be seen. I pause at this.

I believe my Self has a message for me.

Have I ever done this? Indeed, I have. We all have.

Finally, the Gardener positions Himself within a crowd of people. He is within the crowd of people who I feel have inflicted these contractions of offense! I don't want to be near them – they have hurt me. I want to run from them.

She, like the woman who had a divine encounter at the well, braved to enter into the crowd.

The crowd, they bumped into the Gardener. They were not fully present. They did not see with the fullness of the Self. They did not feel with the fullness of their presence. They did not fully encounter Him. They were unaware.

I don't want to just go with the crowd. I want to go deeper. I want to encounter.

These contractions have invited me to go deeper. To encounter.

The woman, this bleeding woman, she went into the crowd, and she was fully present.

She saw the Gardener. She fully encountered Him. She felt Him.

When she felt Him, He felt her touch. He, too, was fully present.

He was available.

If I only go into the crowd, I will only see as the crowd sees.

I need to be willing to go into the crowd.

And I need to be willing to go deeper than the crowd.

Instead of settling on any scraps given to me, I can learn to seek and identify the scraps, the crumbs, the seeds, the moments of value. I can water them and harvest them.

The dripping and the contractions, indications of a labor in progress, did not complete their work to give her the healing she so desired to birth, until she braved to truly be present with the Gardener who gave her the undeserved gift of that grief pregnancy to begin with.

Once she became truly open to His vision of her garden, did it bloom to its greatest.

My friend, whatever your spiritual beliefs are, there is a surrender to accepting that we cannot do it alone. That the best tools and the best people around us still are not enough to manifest the biggest version of our Selves.

This week, I invite you to just contemplate on the little greatness of those around you. Think on the things that you turn to, to feed your soul.

Anything can have good in it. Why shouldn't it? It is found within the garden that is tended by the Great Gardener. But until you have presented your grief pregnancy to the Great Gardener Himself, and let His own hands sculpt the soil, prune the weeds, and touch you, there will be something that will remain unfinished in your labor.

Whatever or whoever you believe your Great Gardener to be, and whatever you may feel toward or about him, it is important to go to him. Other mothers who've endured loss before you hold a great wisdom and have something valuable for you. Others who have seen more of your Great Gardener than you have can share important insights, principles and aspects of him. But they will not deepen your well to the depth it is capable of. They too, can only behold the Great Gardener from a place within their garden. They can speak of the wondrous things they have seen, and you can learn about Him. But learning about Him is not enough. You need to learn *from* Him.

Oh, how often I have neglected to learn You,

and have settled on simply learning about You!

I don't read my Bible to fill time in my day. I don't read my Bible to fill words in my mind, or to accomplish a certain number of pages read or even verses memorized. I read my Bible until I am given a morsel. A tiny crumb of living bread. I hold it on my tongue. I sit with it. It brings me to a place where I am aware that even this entity I am charged with nurturing and disciplining, is not me. Even in the tiniest form of a seed, waited years in my naiveté to implant, this seed is so much bigger than my self.

You may be receiving messages or enduring experiences that indicate that you cannot complete your labor. Enter into your sacred space, and meditate on the possibility of spiritual dystocia in your laboring toward healing.

Ask your Self to speak clearly. Do not let your self fill you with insecurities or shame. Your Self will only speak loving, productive, points of wisdom as your Self shows you how you can keep growing and laboring well.

Preparation

Choose a private place where you feel comfortable and will have no interruptions (turn off your phone, and let others know not to disturb you).

Set aside enough time to do the activity so you do not feel rushed.

Plan to do something relaxing or enjoyable after you have finished the activity.

Try to relax (slow breathing) and clear your mind of other concerns before starting the activity.

The Dare

Listen to the guidance of your Self as you are invited into the presence of the Divine, Great Gardener. Listen to the wisdom as you prepare to experience the birth of healing.

When you are finished listening, journal on your experience.

You can type or handwrite, depending on your preference.

Do not be concerned with spelling, grammar, or punctuation.

Write your account in the first person (use "I" statements).

Write your account in the present tense (as if it is happening right now).

Include as much sensory detail as possible (sights, sounds, smells, textures, etc.)

Include any thoughts and feelings you had at the time.

Even though it may be painful, do not stop yourself from feeling emotions.

Keep writing until your account is complete, even if this takes a while.

When You are Finished

Take time to congratulate yourself on revisiting these feelings.

Treat yourself to something relaxing or enjoyable.

I prepare to meet with my Great Gardener.

I prepare to meet my healing.

Your Sacred Space

___ DARE 32

This week, we are going to get out the scrubbers and our imaginations.

Bring out the bubbles and squeegees.

There is something methodical in cleaning. I love that burst that finds me, that burst of determination and even excitement to get the house clean. Girlfriend, let's nest and prepare our home to be a dwelling place of healing.

We are going to do more than run the vacuum to check this dare off. We are going to spend our morning sacred time taking a walk through our home as we sip our warm sweet snuggle soup of coffee, tea or cocoa together. Observe your home. In what ways is it reflective of your growth toward healing? In what ways has its care been neglected in your grief pregnancy? Let's shape things up around us to reflect the growing that is occurring within us.

Start by choosing one room. I generally prefer my husband's and my bedroom, or the living room. Just, start by choosing one room. Sit in that room or, if he is still sleeping, just sit in your sacred space and imagine the room. Spend time thinking about the things that need organized, the supplies you will need, what things will help fuel you during your work (music, snacks), Can you rearrange the furniture? Can you bring in a piece from somewhere else in the house? Can you pull a piece out? As my thanksgiving list for my husband grows, I select our bedroom and let my imagination find ways to make the room reflect the romance, the fire that burns for my man.

As you begin this project, please be mindful of items that you may have purchased or have gathered in preparation for your baby prior to your pregnancy loss. This dare does not at all suggest to do anything with these items. The decision to change anything about your baby's items needs to be made as a couple, as both parents mutually come to a resolution together.

Preparation

Choose one room in your home that you will open up, air out and refreshen. Gather the supplies you will need. When you are done, journal on the sense of achievement, and of any thoughts you had during the labor.

The Dare

When you are finished cleaning the one room, journal on your experience.

You can type or handwrite, depending on your preference.

Do not be concerned with spelling, grammar, or punctuation.

Write your account in the first person (use "I" statements).

Write your account in the present tense (as if it is happening right now).

Include as much sensory detail as possible (sights, sounds, smells, textures, etc.)

Include any thoughts and feelings you had at the time.

Even though it may be painful, do not stop yourself from

feeling emotions.

Keep writing until your account is complete, even if this takes a while.

When You are Finished

Take time to congratulate yourself on revisiting these feelings.

Treat yourself to something relaxing or enjoyable.

*Where I am indwelled
is beginning to reflect the growing life
indwelling within me.*

Your Sacred Space

__ DARE 33

For this week's dare, I am going to ask you to bask in something you might not have.

Take a milk bath.

I realized, as I neared the birth of my healing, that a thought kept plaguing me like a thorn in my side. With so many experiences of raising a child suddenly incomplete, one of these experiences was in bringing my child to my bosom for nourishment.

It is the reason I found such healing in the professional bra fitting. I needed a woman to wrap her arms around me and tell me just where I was. Yes, the tears streamed down my face as she read that tiny little number to me. I did not hide them. They were cleansing.

This week, I am going to show you how to prepare a milk bath, and I'm going to tell you why it is important to me.

I found a recipe that calls for powdered milk. How fitting. The very first changes that indicate to me that I am possibly pregnant with child include the tingling whirr of mammary glands yawning and beginning their churning of nutrients into milk. After my baby was born via miscarriage, it was as if these sad little women just curled up, sulking.

Dust fell upon my mammary glands.

In the earliest days of my grief pregnancy, I felt so unfamiliar with my body. I felt any truth I had known had abandoned me, and my self certainly filled me with untruths. I began to resent my womanly, motherly breasts for their inability to nourish. I dreaded the presence of the ancient woman flickering the old quilt that releases a crimson flow. What about you? Did you produce breastmilk after your baby was born? Did you donate your breastmilk? Did you dry your milk quickly? I needed desperately to come to a place where I could meet with my feminine self, with my womanly body, and see that I am beautiful. I needed to see that the parts of myself I thought were reserved for nurturing and sustaining a particular life, were nurturing and sustaining life in a way I simply never thought possible. When I completed this dare, when I saw dried up milk coming to life, when I breathed in the beautiful fragrance of lavender, when I dipped my body in and allowed it to be soothed and nurtured, I wept. It was a healing soak.

Beauty from ashes...

Preparation

Gather the supplies needed, and create a time in the evening or in the morning when you can enjoy sacred time soaking in this warm, nurturing, nourishing bath. As you gather the supplies, consider selecting a special aroma (or several) that you can identify with your place in healing.

Supplies:

A jar that seals shut – a lovely idea is to use a glass milk jar, such as from Shatto Farms.
1 cup Epsom salt
1 cup powdered milk
¼ cup baking soda
¼ lavender flowers
4 drops lavender oil

Mix:

Combine all ingredients and store in your jar.
Add ¼ cup of this beautiful mixture to your warm, running bath.

This recipe is found on the web:
http://lifeasmom.com/2012/12/diy-on-a-dime-mix-lavender-milk-bath.html

To learn about essential oils, and to help you in selecting the scent(s) you want to help depict your healing, I would highly recommend visiting the doTERRA website. Here are just a few pieces from their Mood Matrix:

Serenity Calming Blend includes lavender, sweet marjoram, roman chamomile, ylang ylang, sandalwood and vanilla bean extract.

Citrus Bliss Invigorating Blend includes wild orange, lemon, grapefruit, mandarin, bergamot, tangerine, Clementine and vanilla absolute.

Elevation Joyful Blend includes lavandin, tangerine, lemon myrtle, Melissa, ylang ylang, osmanthus and sandalwood.

Balance Grounding Blend includes spruce, rosewood, frankincense, blue tansy and fractionated coconut oil.

Spend some time researching these, and finding local shops within your community where you might sample these to discover the blends, aromas and essential oils that might be best for you.

The Dare

When you are finished with your soak, journal on your experience.

Heidi Faith

Your Sacred Space

__ DARE 34

For this dare, we are going to sing.

A string of noises floats from my soul.

There are some amazingly powerful songs that allow us to enter into the depth of grief, the lyrics bringing us to our pain as if it were still fresh. This particular kind of song holds significance. Just as there are some dares that you will need to revisit to get closer and closer and deeper and deeper into each time, there are parts of our grief that we sometimes don't see until some time later.

For this dare, though, I want you to select a song that is inspiring to you. A song that helps you sweep out the spiritual clutter and that helps to get you inspired as you anticipate meeting your healing.

Maybe do some research into the meaning of the song, its history, its origin. Books such as *Then Sings My Soul: 150 of the World's Greatest Hymn Stories* are such a treasure to snuggle up to and digest.

Consider purchasing the song, in a format that is compatible to your electronics, or as a CD or single. Write out the lyrics in your journal. See if there are other ways to connect with the songwriter, band, or singer.

Allow the lyrics to become a mantra.

This is my benediction.

As you spend your week humming, singing, and thinking on this song, where is your water bottle? Is it near you? Have you tired of drinking water daily? Are you splashing your vocal cords as you stretch them in song? One way I enjoy drinking water, and capturing the sense of consuming living water, is to slice cucumbers and letting them mingle in my bottle.

Preparation

Choose a private place where you feel comfortable and will have no interruptions (turn off your phone, and let others know not to disturb you).

Set aside enough time to do the activity so you do not feel rushed.

Plan to do something relaxing or enjoyable after you have finished the activity.

Try to relax (slow breathing) and clear your mind of other concerns before starting the activity.

The Dare

Listen to the guidance of your Self as you seek wisdom in selecting the right song of your benediction. Ask for the song to be revealed to you in a way that you will know that it is the right song. Be open in your time searching; it is possible that there may be more than one. Consider researching or purchasing something such as *Full Body Blessing: Praying with Movement* by Sparough, Beckman and Fisher.

When you are finished listening, journal on your experience.

You can type or handwrite, depending on your preference.

Do not be concerned with spelling, grammar, or punctuation.

Write your account in the first person (use "I" statements).

Write your account in the present tense (as if it is happening right now).

Include as much sensory detail as possible (sights, sounds, smells, textures, etc.)

Include any thoughts and feelings you had at the time.

Even though it may be painful, do not stop yourself from feeling emotions.

Keep writing until your account is complete, even if this takes a while.

When You are Finished

Take time to congratulate yourself on revisiting these feelings.

Treat yourself to something relaxing or enjoyable.

I find there is something holy in song.
I sing through contractions.

Your Sacred Space

Heidi Faith

__ DARE 35

For this week's dare, I beckon you to become involved in your spiritual community.

Gather in seeking.

It was very difficult for me to attend church regularly while I was pregnant with grief. I felt so confused, so unsettled, about my relationship with the Great Gardener. I wanted to throw a tarp over my landscape and hide from the warmth of the sun. I wanted to shield my eyes from seeing His merciful tears splash through the clouds. Grief somehow weakened the superhero I had believed Him to be. I felt too vulnerable to begin again, exploring and identifying and trusting Him.

Through my grief pregnancy, I grew a hunger, though. A hunger to know, to really know, what happened to my child. More than the why or the how, I wanted to know *what now?* I needed to know.

I heard the whisper of my Self, and, feeling so misunderstood by the world around me, I began to enter into my sacred space and allow my Self the room to talk freely with me. Eventually, the hunger grew, to be in the place where I knew a trusted leader could lead me to a mantra, could lead me to a morsel of the living bread.

I had so many big feelings about my relationship with my Great Gardener, that just driving on the paving in front of the church brought anxiety. Standing, within a congregation of believers, within a community of people, us, a bouquet of wild flowers, waving to the winds of the Holy Spirit blowing kisses through our outreached hands, our open pours, filling our wells with fresh clean water, I burst into tears. The salt of anger, rejection, shame, resentment, despair, and longing all brimmed over and poured over me. Sabbath after Sabbath, I cleansed my Self this way.

As we shake each other's hands and say "Good morning" before finding our seats, we could rest, knowing that as we are in this place for spiritual bread, so too are those around us.

I sometimes feel that God, the Great Gardener of my soul, prunes and cuts too deeply. I don't think He does it carelessly, I feel He is very present and very aware of His work, but alas, I feel sometimes He cuts to the quick. My miscarriage – my baby had a perfectly fine place to grow. Why did He uproot this growth? I am submissive to His hands and beg Him to prune gently. Don't leave this stretch of land so raw!

What has happened since He has taken this perfectly fine life? My physical form has ached and yearned for nurturance because of the spiritual growth that has taken place. And in this journey, I have discovered that my spiritual growth too, needs to be fed.

The seed comes from somewhere, from a place too hidden and marvelous for my frail earthen eyes to see. As my soul rises and reaches to the Gardener, waving my hands, begging for a drink, I sense my child's soul is with Him. In fact, I mostly sense that my child is too distracted looking at beautiful, magnificent things to even put presence into my outstretched hands. His physical form is still bringing life, after all. His dismissive glance down at my mortal misunderstandings fills me with confirmation that I am being led into a sacred journey to resemble this magnificence that I can't even see but that somehow, I do behold.

I am drawn to a parable of a sower and a seed:

A farmer went out to sow his seed. As he was scattering the seed, some fell along the path, and the birds came and ate it up. Some fell on rocky places, where it did not have much soil. It sprang up quickly, because the soil was shallow. But when the sun came up, the plants were scorched, and they withered because they had no root. Other seed fell among thorns, which grew up and choked the plants. Still other seed fell on good soil, where it produced a crop – a hundred, sixty or thirty times what was sown.
– Matthew 13:3-8

I contemplate on this message. I hold it silently, as I feel that stirring within telling me there is much to harvest from these words.

Fell along the path – I dwell on the thought, and, it reminds me of ectopic pregnancy.

Rocky places, with little soil – this draws into my mind hormonal complications that prevent a deep embedding of the baby into mother's endometrium.

Falling among thorns – images float into my mind of so many obstacles parents face in fertility, such as physical growths or scars that get in the way.

As I find these thoughts, a deep cry escapes me, for the hundreds of thousands of families who have braved to reach out to share their stories and their experiences.

What morsel of living bread, of hope, could possibly be uncovered through this passage?

I spend the time I need to, weeping, the tears of respect, reverence and love for these families outpouring from the deepest part of my well, where the salt has settled below.

When I have honored these families until exhaustion, I quiet myself to listen for the answer to my cry.

I am moved to the physical process of human fertilization. I see a very scientific process through a microscopic lens that allows me to travel with man's seed, the smallest part that is of him but not him, and I see, I see the millions of swooshing sperm, wriggling, inching, crawling, through the secret tunnel that fits them so well, a fallopian tube. The cilia wave and cheer in delight as they welcome these guests through the corridor and usher them to meet her.

There she is, this beautiful bride, adorned in white. The momentum builds, the excitement mounts, as they each rush to woo her and insist that they are most worthy.

In the physical process of conception, a great many of the man's seeds stop right there, along the path. Over the next several hours, these seeds slide down the hillside where the woman finds them, dripped onto her panties.

My Self poses a question for me to ponder:

If the Great Gardener broadcasts His seeds in this way, what seeds are lost when the seed of the child is the one that grows to ripeness within his mother's womb?

The question confuses my frail mind, and so I dwell on it as I think on the families who I have been present with during the births of their living children.

Has the attention, nurturance and discipline given in tending to the growth of the child seed ever abandoned care for the Self seed?

I taste the rust of ancient wisdom as my Self brings a truth from the depths:

Every time the Great Gardener spreads the seed of the child, He too spreads the seed of Self.

Every child seed, and every Self seed, is subjected to the

potential elements of falling along the path, of falling along rocky places with little soil, and of falling among thorns.

Contemplatively, I review the parable in this light.

I discover promises embedded within the words.

There is never anything wrong with the Great Gardener's seed. There is never anything wrong with the soil of my soul. Once I identify that the seed of Self has been implanted, once I learn to nurture it and discipline it as needed, it will produce a crop.

It is from within my grief pregnancy, it is from the loss of my child, that I have come to identify this seed of Self. My self hisses an accusatory thought, *"Did I need the one to perish for me to see the other?"* My soul groans as my earthly mind is just too small to know. I don't know why I entered into this grief pregnancy. I release the want to know. I remain present, now, here, within it. It is the way I know to ensure tending to this growing life within.

I want my Self to resemble my child.

I want my landscape to resemble

my Great Gardener.

I want the spiritual gifts of my child

and of my Self

to grow to all they can be.

I desire to participate in the laboring

of the Great Gardener of my soul.

Preparation

Decide on a local temple or other spiritual education and worship center. Prepare for attending, by researching in advance their beliefs, their service times, their dress code, and anything else you may need to know.

If you are already engaged in a spiritual center, explore this week additional ways you might get involved. Is there a women's group? Does your spiritual leader have resources specific to parental bereavement that you could explore? Is there an activity taking place that you could simply help with in some way?

The Dare

After you have carefully, mindfully and prayerfully selected a spiritual center, attend a worship service. Listen for your mantra.

When you are finished listening, back at home in your sacred space, journal on your experience.

You can type or handwrite, depending on your preference.

Do not be concerned with spelling, grammar, or punctuation.

Write your account in the first person (use "I" statements).

Write your account in the present tense (as if it is happening right now).

Include as much sensory detail as possible (sights, sounds, smells, textures, etc.)

Include any thoughts and feelings you had at the time.

Even though it may be painful, do not stop yourself from feeling emotions.

Keep writing until your account is complete, even if this takes a while.

When You are Finished

Take time to congratulate yourself on revisiting these feelings.

Treat yourself to something relaxing or enjoyable.

My child is exploring heights of Truth
that I can't even imagine
until I let my Self grow tall enough to
glimpse, and capture the vision for me.

Heidi Faith

Your Sacred Space

__ DARE 36

This week, I'm going to challenge you to give.

Giving...

Giving can be painful to do, especially when we feel we have lost so much.

I look around my home. I have recently taken on the dare of really entering into, cleaning out and opening up a room in my home. I have enjoyed it so entirely that the endorphins take momentum and I move into another space in my home to do the same. In the process, I have rearranged, exchanged and removed some items of furniture, dishes, and other things. They have sat in a pile in my garage, as if to say, "We do have value, we are not trash, but we do not find place in the new space here."

I call my church, I read the newspaper, I email local charities and organizations to find a new home where the value in these pieces will be found.

There is a treasure to harvest in the tilling of your tangible resources, brushing off the dirt and studying the fruits. Have you found it? It is the treasure of discovering that you behold abundant fruit. As you select that which is appropriate to gift to others, you are gardening your home, pruning even the branches that still provide. And when you are finished, you still possess the things of greatest value and potential to serve you.

Why does the vinedresser prune even those branches that do bear fruit? This question beckons me to allow it to become my mantra during my work of giving.

Preparation

Decide on at least one item that you can give or share with others. Do not give anything that was part of your gathering in preparation for your child, unless you have the mutual consent from your husband to do so. Your item can be a piece of furniture such as a chair or lamp, it can be a craft or something you can create or cook, or it can be a small portion of your money. When giving money, consider the cause and if it aligns well with your labor of growing your Self. Charities to consider may include St. Jude's Children's Hospital, Salvation Army, Ronald McDonald House, or, you may feel led to begin contributing a tithe or giving an offering at your spiritual center.

The Dare

Be mindful and present during the laboring process of gifting something that still holds some value to another. When you have finished this task, journal on the experience.

You can type or handwrite, depending on your preference.

Do not be concerned with spelling, grammar, or punctuation.

Write your account in the first person (use "I" statements).

Write your account in the present tense (as if it is happening right now).

Include as much sensory detail as possible (sights, sounds, smells, textures, etc.)

Include any thoughts and feelings you had at the time.

Even though it may be painful, do not stop yourself from feeling emotions.

Keep writing until your account is complete, even if this takes a while.

When You are Finished

Take time to congratulate yourself on revisiting these feelings.

Treat yourself to something relaxing or enjoyable.

In giving, I find that I receive.

Your Sacred Space

Heidi Faith

__ DARE 37

This week, I am going to dare you to indulge and care for your external landscape.

Indulge in feminine luxury.

"Luxury" is a word that even just sounds luxurious, doesn't it? It conjures feelings of extravagance, it brings images of deep satisfaction, but as it lingers, it brings a sense of wastefulness, selfishness, and of really not being needed.

I confront these messages that denounce the beauty and worth of luxury. And in my stillness, I find that some luxury is, in fact, important.

It is in disciplining the luxury that prevents it from festering into wastefulness that feeds the self and grows selfishness.

So this week, we are going to nurture our desire for luxury. Later, we will discipline it.

This week, consider your budget, and determine a practical allowance for a little indulgence. Here are some suggested ideas, all within various budgets:

Visit a spa. This might be an eyebrow waxing, a back massage, or a warm, wrap massage. You might try one tanning session, and as you contemplate that option, evaluate the time you've enjoyed lately in the sunshine. During the planning to complete this dare, you might determine to hold some of your sacred space outdoors, with a comfortable blanket and shorts, to feel the adoring kiss of the sun. Visit spa websites to determine pricing – you will be delighted to see that many of these services are affordable.

Get a professional nail service. I recommend a pedicure over a manicure, but both are wonderful. Again, research ahead of time, looking for photos of the facility and customer reviews. Even walk in and just see what some of the facilities look like and have to offer. You are looking for a business that sets a tone of relaxation and indulgence. If the business gives too cramped of a feeling, or is located in a place of high retail traffic such as a mall or in a chain store, you should keep searching.

Get a professional hair washing. Yes, you can set an appointment just for a hair washing. There is something surrendering in letting her dip your head back into the sink, letting her guide you so that you don't injure your head on the lip of the ceramic bowl. The invigorating sensations of her fingers stimulating your scalp and the water cleaning your hair follicles is a delight. Hair loss is common after the birth of a child, and you might have experienced this, particularly in the earliest days in your grief pregnancy. Consider a trim, to freshen up the ends that divide and open up room for richer growth.

You can even make a homemade facial peel or scrub. I love the sensation of removing the old face and revealing a fresh, radiant presence. Doing a little research, you can even make one that is edible, to make it more fun.

Have you continued planning your ladies slumber party? You might consider this week's assignment as a trial to determine an additional activity to include with your girlfriends.

Preparation

Spend time evaluating your desires in completing this dare, and in researching the best businesses to serve you, and in determining the most appropriate budget.

The Dare

Be mindful and present during the experience of submitting to the gentle touch of a professional serving you. Be mindful and present during the experiences of surrender, of relaxation, of pleasure, of delight. When you are finished and return to your sacred space, dwell on these sensations. Journal your experience.

You can type or handwrite, depending on your preference.

Do not be concerned with spelling, grammar, or punctuation.

Write your account in the first person (use "I" statements).

Write your account in the present tense (as if it is happening right now).

Include as much sensory detail as possible (sights, sounds, smells, textures, etc.)

Include any thoughts and feelings you had at the time.

Even though it may be painful, do not stop yourself from feeling emotions.

Keep writing until your account is complete, even if this takes a while.

When You are Finished

Take time to congratulate yourself on revisiting these feelings.

Treat yourself to something relaxing or enjoyable

I am treated as if I am beautiful,

and it relaxes me.

I am beautiful. I am valuable.

Your Sacred Space

__ DARE 38

This dare calls you into movement.

Get moving!

We've had a couple of dares where we've been outdoors. We went for an intentional walk, we've painted with mud, and last week's dare might have encouraged you to get out into the sunshine. As you looked at activities you might enjoy, by now you should be engaged in one, and it might be brisk walking or physically working out.

The most optimum of sensory experiences for this dare would include being outdoors, alone, with a device that plays your special song, your invocation to healing, on a warm, sunny day.

Dressed in sturdy sneakers and loose, comfortable clothes, you can begin this dare by entering into a special wilderness, much like the intentional walk you took in days passed. As you become relaxed and feeling safe in this place, when you are ready, I want you to play your song, and I want you to use your body to paint the strokes of the Great Gardener in His laboring over your soul.

Standing, feet comfortably apart, hold your arms in a ballet first position, as a farmer holding a very large bag of his seeds.

Search the ground before you with artistic deliberation, determining that the landscape is well. Stamp and stomp your feet atop the earth, waking it, disciplining it, shaping it, preparing it for growth. Alternate pressing the points of your toes into the ground, as if you are opening up spaces for the seeds to fill.

Spreading your arms open now into a ballet second position, imagine sprinkling this seeds onto the good soil.

In an Arabesque type form, imagine your feminine mothering sprinkling seeds of life into Mother Earth, as if the two of you are dear sisters or close womanly relatives passing a treasured recipe or heirloom to one another.

I gift Mother Earth with seeds of Self.

In ballet fourth position, imagine you are holding your own burlap of seeds. You hold them to your bosom, you warm them with your heart. You see that you are so much smaller than your Great Gardener, but you delight in being able to mimic His work. You dare to toss a handful of seeds over your shoulder. You do not care less about these seeds, in fact it is possible that you care about them more – at least, you certainly pause and fill the moment with intention and with prayer. These seeds, you will let go. You will not chart their height over time. These seeds, you surrender to the process of life. These seeds are good. The soil is good. You entrust that if these seeds do not produce fruit, they will, in some way, lead another special soul to your harvest.

I go back to the parable of the farmer and the seeds. I know that birds were a part of the process. As the laboring enters a transitional phase, the seeds nourished life in a whole new, unexpected way. They satisfied the birds. The meager droplets of their moisture were swallowed into the water cycle, invited into this transition by the warmth of the sun. I surrender to the knowledge and to the power of my little greatness.

In motion, swaying, stooping and stretching, my dance is prayer.

I labor over my seeds and know that they
will produce a harvest of love.
The life these seeds bare resembles my child.
They are my Self.

Preparation

Gather supplies needed: sturdy shoes, comfortable clothes, your water bottle, your music, a blanket and your journal.

The Dare

Enter into your outdoor space. Perform your spiritual dance. When you are finished, rest on your blanket and journal your experience.

You can type or handwrite, depending on your preference.

Do not be concerned with spelling, grammar, or punctuation.

Write your account in the first person (use "I" statements).

Write your account in the present tense (as if it is happening right now).

Include as much sensory detail as possible (sights, sounds, smells, textures, etc.)

Include any thoughts and feelings you had at the time.

Even though it may be painful, do not stop yourself from feeling emotions.

Keep writing until your account is complete, even if this takes a while.

When You are Finished

Take time to congratulate yourself on revisiting these feelings.

Treat yourself to something relaxing or enjoyable

I surrender to the knowledge and to the

power

of my little greatness.

Your Sacred Space

Heidi Faith

__ DARE 39

So many times I would wonder, "Is this the end, or is this just the beginning" when I would hear my Self reply,

This is both.

The birth of healing is a lot like the beginning of grief – some pains resemble the beginning, and may make you wonder just how far you've really come.

Take pause, and give this statement some time to be with you.

Have you begun to forget any particular things about your child? While some things will stand out in significance to you, you will find that you perhaps have clasped to these things and have inadvertently let other things go. Some mothers hold a very powerful sense, a seemingly fresh sense of grief, around their baby's due date. Perhaps this is in exchange for remembering what brand of pregnancy test used to determine the pregnancy. What hair clip you wore when you first discovered crimson in your panties may be long forgotten. The make and model of the cars that were parked around you may elude your memory as you call into your mind leaving the doctor's office, devastated at hearing that your child is no longer alive.

When a baby dies, even if he dies still within you, changes to his physical form happen rapidly. Many families fear that these changes will inhibit them from basking in the wonder of the creation of their child, and find that they do not nearly as much as they feared. However, while we can help to chill their physical form, or if they are very tiny, submerge their physical form in salted water, we soon meet the realization that these changes are simply outside of our control. The Great Gardener has already determined that each of us vessels will live, that we will nourish one another in some way. This divine law is outside of our grasp to control or change. We simply find our little greatness and grow to embrace it.

It is the same in our earthly minds. A divine law gardens our minds, and while we too have a responsibility and a privilege to participate as an arborist of our minds, ultimately the ancient wisdom of the Great Gardener reigns more supreme than our meager strain of determination. In short, we cannot will ourselves to remember everything. In our minds, as in our souls, a space is made for bigger growth. We are called to see our child in a bigger way. We are called to see our motherhood in a bigger way.

Release the slipping grasp to cling to memories or visions that glimpse of the smallness of your child, of the frailty of his potential, of the cessation of his meaning, of the sense of even losing him whatsoever.

Your child's life, neither physically nor spiritually, has come to an end. Rather, a momentum has built, a climax is unfolding, and a great transition is being witnessed and experienced.

The reasons for your child's death are both physical and spiritual, and although I know neither reason, both hold opportunities for you to discover seeds, for you to nurture them, and for you to discipline them. I don't know why you are on the landscape you are on, but I call to you from mine, from a place where I felt cold, naked, abandoned, where I felt cut to the quick. I felt whipped by the winds of the Holy Spirit and I felt scorched by the furnace of God. I felt empty, and I felt like I needed cover.

I call to you, a promise, that you have been given seeds. I promise you will find them, if you quiet your self to look. I promise that if you nurture these seeds, and if you discipline these seeds, that they will grow. Be encouraged, that you do not need yet to know how to grow this new life, or even what to fully expect it to look like. Be still. Listen. The Great Gardener will show you how.

Take time in your sacred space to journal how some pains you are facing, some encounters you are enduring for the first time, how they resemble the beginning, how they challenge you and try to belittle your growth.

See how the farmer waits for the land to yield its valuable crop from the earth, being patient with it until it receives the early and the late rains. You also must be patient. Strengthen your hearts, for the coming of the Lord is near. – James 5:7-8

This week, consider purchasing or creating a focal point. It should be an item that isn't just symbolic of your child, but also symbolic of how the knowledge of being this child's mother has grown you.

I think of that empty feeling I once had that seemed to just ache of hollowness. I remember feeling so violently exposed. I needed to take cover, I needed to rest my head. I am led to the psalms, songs of those long before me who also found their painful path to trading in their watering jars for wells.

Be my rock of refuge, to which I can always go; give the command to save me, for you are my rock and my fortress. Deliver me, my God. From birth I have relied on you. –Psalm 71:3-6

These few verses capture me, and at first I don't know why. I hold them on my lips and move them around with my tongue. I wait and listen and chew on them.

A rock, a blessed rock, can deliver. A rock, a blessed rock, was revisited and relied upon since birth.

Have you purchased a headstone for your child?

Have you selected a special stone – perhaps from any of your sacred outings – and brought it home with you? Consider finding a special stone, and placing it in a place in your back yard, creating a place that invites you to sit Burmese on the growing grass around it and know that it is symbolic of the God who can deliver your healing.

One version of this special stone may be in purchasing a special piece of jewelry that holds your child's birthstone.

When you become a mother, it is not as much of a life leaving you, as a life entering you. As you discover that this life has entered you, you then enter into a new life.

I implore you to see that you are in this new life.

You are to mother the seed you believe is lost by mothering the seeds within.

One way that I find successful in assuring me that I do in fact have an eternal life within me, and that I can even engage in this holy life now, is to empty of the things I do know, to find what, if anything, is left.

It seems there was a bigger reason for feeling so empty after my baby had died and was born.

I was being invited to enter into this emptiness to identify its purpose. Not the reasons for my child's death, mind you, but the reasons for the emptiness I held.

To enter into this emptiness, this dare calls you to something known as fasting, although what takes place is quite the opposite.

The best way to complete this dare is through wise preparation.

Enter into your sacred space, and present your Self with the proposition of refraining from eating any food for one day. Allow all of the reasons for the difficulty of this task to come forward.

Examine the days ahead on your calendar, and decide if one day is more available for your fast. Perhaps it is a day you will not have to drive or work, but can remain home. Anticipate what you believe will be the best, most nutritious meal to eat before bed the night before, and what the best, most nutritious meal will be to eat as evening sets on the day of your fast, being sure to read and follow the instructions below.

Prepare and plan for the day of your fast.

We are going to make what is called a beggars bowl, and we will use our gratitude jar to do so.

On the morning of your fast, empty the jar of love notes to your Self.

For one day, from your early morning sacred time until the sun has gone down, refrain from consuming any food whatsoever. If you have health or medical conditions which pose serious challenges to fasting for the entire day, consider holding any sort of variation of the Daniel fast.

You can and should drink water as desired throughout the time of your fast.

Every time your stomach grumbles, voicing its complaint and its yearning for food, remember how frail your physical form is. Remember how often you tend to it without putting presence into the act. Remember how you have fed it junk that did not nourish it. Sip your cleansing water.

There is a space, an emptiness, and you are sensing it and feeling it. You are cleansing it.

Your cravings try to interrupt you but with each passing hour, you are disciplining your self while nurturing your Self. You hold your thoughts captive.

Wrap your hands around your beggars bowl.

Hold your palms around it until you feel a warmth growing.

Ask your Self to fill this jar with living water, with affirmations of your little greatness.

Peer down into your beggars bowl as the yearnings of your flesh seem unbearable. Drink up the words of love you are given, the encouragement, the strength you find.

You are little. And you are great.

At the end of your day, consume only enough food that will fit within your beggars bowl.

After your meal, journal on your experience.

*There is more in me than
I have once made room for.
I don't have to understand
or even accept the reasons given to me
for my child's death,
while embracing that it has only been through
his death that I have discovered this vast space
for growth. I behold plenty of landscape as I
tend to this new, mysterious, beautiful garden.*

My Sacred Space

Heidi Faith

__ DARE 40

You've been patient. You've been diligent. You've witnessed the toiling and you've entered into laboring with presence. Still, you don't find that you've truly given birth to healing.

What are my options?

It's OK to say you need more help than what you've been given.

This book has only been a guide. I am a landscape, a mere enfleshed seed. I see my great big gardener and have tried to mimic his movements, but I cannot breathe a soul into a vessel. I cannot speak intention and birth your healing and gift it to you.

I am sorry.

There is more nurturing, more disciplining, in your grief pregnancy. Perhaps this is a place to determine what other tools there are to help in this labor.

Going on an "oxytocin scavenger hunt" can be one fun way

to try some things that bring you pleasure, as you then review and redo some of the dares in this book. Oxtocin is a hormone that not only allows for loving feelings to proliferate, but even help to prepare your soul's landscape for healing.

Speaking privately with a trusted friend, possibly one who has also endured pregnancy and infant loss, is an option.

Arranging a meeting with a wise mentor, such as a pastor, is an excellent idea.

There are local, national and global resources for long term support listed at stillbirthday; resources like MEND.

Possibly considering a session with a counselor will prove to open up more options for you to mindfully, carefully, and prayerfully consider, such as medications or other therapies.

These things will not replace your participation in your labor. These things will instead serve to attempt to magnify the results of your own efforts. You will still need to labor through the transition.

You will still need to learn the little greatness that you are.

Thank you for lovingly embracing me as I am while the murky layers of my many shortcomings are slowly transformed in love. – Joyce Rupp in Prayers for Sophia

May I believe the things that are true about me, no matter how wonderful they are. -Macrina Wiederkehr

What is it like, to give birth to healing?

How will I know when I have?

Does it mean I won't have grief anymore?

These are questions that we all ask, and in fear of losing the little we have, we fear opening our Selves to receiving more.

As you find healing, you will still miss your child.

As you find healing, you will still think of him and long for him.

As you behold your healing, yes, you will still have grief, in much the same way a mother beholds her naked newborn but still carries within her real traces of his physical presence, for eternity.

When you find healing, the starving strikes of hunger for him begin to be softened with affirmations of how he has grown in the world and how he has grown in you.

When you find healing, you may silently find annoyance that your loved ones don't bring you back to the memories of your child (they stop mentioning the experience), but you can identify that this void is filled with affirmations of how you have grown in your new life.

When you behold healing, you will find reverence for your child's little greatness, for your own little greatness, and for the undeserved gift that the two are eternally, physically, and spiritually, inseparable.

When you trust healing, you will find magnificent wonder in the process of your labor in presenting the biggest version of your Self as you embed into the womb of Mother Earth on a day that is coming yet which we know not exactly when.

When you embrace healing, you will find joy in the labor of presenting the biggest version of your Self to your child on a day that is coming yet which we know not exactly when.

I weep, full of humility and thankfulness,
of surrender and of conviction.
I am in a new place.   I have healing.

My Sacred Space

Heidi Faith

AFTER HEALING IS BORN

You know that as you labored and gave birth to your child, that the work wasn't finished. You recall the feeling of the earliest weeks, when the support, validation and attention began to wane. It appeared as if the story had ended, the movie theatre had cleared, the book had been shut, when the climax had reached.

There was then and is now much more to the story. Something has ended, and yet something has begun.

Your work is yet unfinished.

Your garden of Self may be big and wide enough for you to stroll through, and may provide satisfying fruit to nourish the world, but you still need to observe your Great Gardener in nurturing and in disciplining.

I will be bereaved eternally, as I am a mother eternally. I am a mother whose water jar was taken, and who humbly understood the need to trade it to become a well. I learned the importance of surrendering my water jar, even though it was taken. The seed of gestation did not grow my child in the way that I thought, hoped for and planned for. The seed of life I ached to hear giggle, I do not have the ears in this frail earthly vessel to hear.

My self often hisses accusations of belittlement and inconsequence as I toil in my garden. Alas, I daily find a weed of dishonesty taunting me and provoking me to forget my little greatness, and the responsibility I have to mother my child by surrendering my Self to the nurturance and the discipline it requires to grow to be the biggest version it can be.

I mend the space after my pregnancy and infant loss by allowing it to be filled with my child's greatest physical and spiritual potential.

Growing my Self to all it can be, is the most honoring way to mother my child.

The Great Gardener trains me to become a part of this process.

His wisdom is ancient and His plans for me and my child are eternal.

Your Sacred Space

.

ABOUT THE AUTHOR

For ten years Heidi Faith counseled at-risk and abused teens, guiding them in a special way because she once was one. In her first pregnancy she discovered the seed of Self, and switched professions to birth support, where she spent years guiding families through the experiences of pregnancy, labor and childbirth. The birth of her fourth child embedded within her a desire to support families enduring pregnancy and infant loss, and called her to see that the Self, implanted so long ago, needed her mothering, her nurturing and her discipline.

It was in creating stillbirthday that Heidi came to hear the words of her soul, speak the truth of the Invisible Pregnancy.

If you are pregnant with child, are pregnant with grief, with both, or ever have been pregnant with either, please visit *www.stillbirthday.com*.

What I was told was a mere pregnancy loss is still a birthday, a day that marks a sacred end and a sacred beginning, and I am still and will eternally be a mother, to child and to grief. Come, allow me to guide you, with tools, wisdom and love for both.

Made in the USA
Middletown, DE
12 April 2015